Escape Bedside Burnout

The Complete Guide to Building a Six-Figure Legal Nurse Consulting Practice

Etta Alison Knapp

This book is designed to provide information and guidance about legal nurse consulting as a career option. It is sold with the understanding that the author and publisher are not engaged in rendering legal, medical, accounting, or other professional services. If legal advice or other expert assistance is required, the services of a competent professional should be sought.

The information contained in this book is based on the author's experience and research as of the publication date. The legal nurse consulting field, healthcare regulations, legal requirements, and professional standards are subject to change. Readers should verify current requirements and seek appropriate professional guidance before making career or business decisions.

This book is intended for educational and informational purposes only. The content is not intended to replace formal education, certification programs, or professional training required for legal nurse consulting practice. Readers should pursue appropriate education, certification, and licensing as required by their jurisdiction and intended practice area.

While this book contains strategies and advice that have worked for many legal nurse consultants, there is no guarantee that these methods will produce successful results for every reader. Success in legal nurse consulting depends on numerous factors including individual skills, market conditions, economic factors, and professional effort that are beyond the author's control.

The author and publisher make no representations or warranties regarding the potential income, success, or outcomes that may result from implementing the strategies described in this book. Past performance and examples cited do not guarantee future results.

The business strategies, financial planning advice, and investment recommendations contained in this book are general in nature and may not be suitable for every individual's circumstances. Readers should consult with qualified business advisors, accountants, attorneys, and financial planners before making business decisions or investments based on information in this book.

Tax laws, business regulations, and licensing requirements vary by jurisdiction and change frequently. The author and publisher are not responsible for any financial losses or legal consequences resulting from business decisions made based on information in this book.

Professional liability and risk management requirements vary by state, practice type, and individual circumstances.

Readers should consult with qualified insurance professionals, attorneys, and risk management experts to determine appropriate coverage and compliance requirements for their specific practice situations.

To the fullest extent permitted by law, the author and publisher shall not be liable for any damages, including but not limited to, direct, indirect, incidental, consequential, or punitive damages arising from the use of this book or the inability to use information contained herein, even if the author or publisher has been advised of the possibility of such damages.

In no event shall the total liability of the author and publisher exceed the purchase price of this book.

By using this book, readers agree to indemnify and hold harmless the author and publisher from any claims, damages, losses, or expenses (including attorney fees) arising from their use of the information contained herein or any actions taken based on such information.

By reading and using this book, you acknowledge that you have read, understood, and agree to be bound by this disclaimer in its entirety. If you do not agree with any part of this disclaimer, you should not use the information contained in this book.

ISBN: 978-1-7642235-0-8

Isohan Publishing

Table of Contents

Chapter 1: The LNC Revolution - Why Now Is Your Time

The healthcare industry stands at a crossroads where nursing expertise meets legal necessity, creating an unprecedented opportunity for nurses ready to step beyond traditional bedside roles. You possess something attorneys desperately need but cannot obtain elsewhere: the clinical knowledge to bridge medicine and law in ways that make or break million-dollar cases.

This shift represents more than career change—it's professional transformation driven by fundamental changes in how legal cases require medical interpretation. Every medical malpractice lawsuit, every personal injury claim, every workers' compensation case needs someone who understands both the clinical realities of patient care and the evidentiary requirements of legal proceedings. That someone could be you.

The $20 Billion Legal Consulting Boom and Nurse Opportunity

Legal consulting services have exploded into a $20 billion industry projected to reach unprecedented heights by 2033[1]. This growth stems from increasingly complex healthcare litigation requiring specialized medical knowledge that traditional legal professionals simply cannot provide. Attorneys find themselves drowning in medical records they cannot interpret, facing expert witnesses they cannot properly prepare, and missing critical clinical insights that determine case outcomes.

The numbers tell a compelling story. Over 1.3 million attorneys practice in the United States, yet fewer than 5,000 certified legal nurse consultants serve this massive market[2]. This shortage creates extraordinary opportunity for nurses willing to develop the skills attorneys value most: the ability to translate medical complexity into clear, actionable legal strategy.

Consider the case of Maria Rodriguez, a 15-year ICU veteran who made the transition in 2019. Her first major case involved a medication error that resulted in patient death. The plaintiff's attorney had been struggling for months to understand the complex interaction between multiple medications, the patient's underlying conditions, and the hospital's protocols. Maria's analysis revealed the critical error: a miscommunication during shift change that led to double-dosing of a cardiac medication. Her work directly contributed to a $2.8 million settlement, earning her a $15,000 fee for three weeks of part-time analysis work.

Another success story comes from David Chen, an emergency department nurse who specialized in trauma cases. His clinical experience with motorcycle accidents made him invaluable to personal injury attorneys handling similar cases. David's understanding of injury patterns, treatment protocols, and long-term prognosis helped attorneys build stronger cases. Within two years, he built a practice generating over $180,000 annually while working fewer hours than his hospital job required.

The legal industry's desperation for medical expertise manifests in multiple ways. Insurance companies pay premium rates for nurses who can identify fraudulent claims by recognizing inconsistencies between reported injuries and documented treatment. Law firms handling class-action pharmaceutical litigation need nurses who understand drug mechanisms, side effect profiles, and clinical trial protocols. Government agencies investigating healthcare fraud rely on nurses who can spot billing irregularities and care deficiencies that indicate systematic problems.

This demand creates multiple revenue streams for skilled legal nurse consultants. Beyond traditional case analysis, opportunities include expert witness testimony, medical record organization, healthcare policy consulting, and litigation support services. Each avenue offers different compensation structures and time commitments, allowing you to build a practice that fits your lifestyle and financial goals.

Geographic Hotspots and Remote Work Advantages

Location dramatically influences earning potential and opportunity availability in legal nurse consulting. **Washington state leads compensation** with average annual salaries reaching $96,429 for employed legal nurse consultants[3]. New York follows closely at $91,272, while California offers $89,156. These figures reflect both higher costs of living and greater concentration of complex litigation requiring specialized medical expertise.

However, malpractice activity patterns reveal different opportunities. **New York dominates total malpractice payouts** with $372.39 million across 659 claims in 2024[4]. Florida shows the highest claim volume with 670 cases, though individual settlements average lower. Texas, Pennsylvania, and Illinois round out the top five states for malpractice activity, each representing significant markets for legal nurse consulting services.

The geographic concentration creates strategic advantages for nurses willing to work remotely. Sarah Martinez, a former OR nurse in rural Montana, built her practice serving law firms in New York and California through virtual consultations and electronic record review. Her lower overhead costs combined with premium market rates allowed her to achieve six-figure income while maintaining small-town lifestyle. She explains: "Attorneys don't care where I live. They care about the quality of my analysis and my ability to explain complex surgical procedures in ways juries understand."

Post-pandemic remote work acceptance has permanently changed legal practice norms. Virtual depositions, once rare exceptions, now represent standard procedure for many firms. Electronic record sharing, secure video conferencing, and cloud-based case management systems enable legal nurse consultants to serve clients nationwide without geographic limitations.

This shift particularly benefits nurses in lower-cost areas who can access higher-paying markets. A nurse in Alabama can command New York rates while maintaining Alabama living costs, dramatically improving earning potential. Rural nurses gain access to specialized case types rarely seen in their local markets, allowing expertise development that would be impossible through local opportunities alone.

Salary Comparison: $93K RN vs $150K+ LNC Potential

The financial transformation from registered nurse to legal nurse consultant represents one of nursing's most significant earning opportunities. **Median RN salary nationwide reaches $93,600 annually[5]**, but this figure masks the reality of demanding schedules, mandatory overtime, and limited advancement opportunities that define hospital nursing.

Legal nurse consulting offers dramatically different compensation structures. **Independent consultants command $125-175 per hour** for case analysis work[6]. Expert witness testimony rates range from $250-400 per hour, with court appearances often requiring full-day commitments paid at premium rates. Successful independent practitioners regularly achieve $150,000-250,000 in annual revenue, with top performers exceeding $300,000.

Jennifer Thompson's transition illustrates this potential. As a pediatric ICU nurse in Chicago, she earned $78,000 annually working 12-hour shifts with frequent overtime. The emotional toll of losing young patients, combined with understaffing and increasing administrative burdens, led her to explore alternatives. After completing legal nurse consultant training, she began accepting cases involving pediatric malpractice and medical device failures.

Her first year generated $45,000 in consulting fees while maintaining her hospital position part-time. By year two, legal nurse consulting income reached $89,000, allowing her to leave bedside nursing entirely. Year three brought $156,000 in revenue from just 28 hours per week of work. Jennifer notes: "I still use my nursing knowledge every day, but instead of being physically and emotionally drained, I feel intellectually challenged and professionally valued."

The compensation structure favors expertise over time investment. While hospitals pay nurses for hours worked regardless of patient acuity or outcomes, legal consulting rewards knowledge, analysis quality, and case impact. A single high-value case analysis might generate $10,000-15,000 in fees for work completed over several weeks at your own pace.

Employee positions in legal nurse consulting also offer superior compensation compared to traditional nursing roles. **Insurance companies pay $65,000-85,000 for claims review nurses[7]**, positions that typically involve regular business hours, no weekends or holidays, and comprehensive benefits packages. Law firms employ legal nurse consultants at $70,000-95,000 annually, with bonus structures tied to case outcomes and client satisfaction.

Beyond base compensation, legal nurse consulting offers expense deduction opportunities unavailable to employed nurses. Home office expenses, professional development costs, travel to depositions, and specialized software purchases become tax-deductible business expenses, effectively increasing take-home income.

Post-COVID Permanent Changes in Legal Practice

The COVID-19 pandemic accelerated legal industry technological adoption by decades, creating permanent changes that benefit legal nurse consultants. **Virtual depositions, once rare exceptions, became standard practice overnight[8]**. This shift eliminated geographic barriers that previously limited nurse consultant opportunities to local markets.

Before 2020, most depositions required physical presence in attorney offices or court facilities. This limitation forced legal nurse consultants to focus on nearby cases or incur significant travel expenses for out-of-state opportunities. The pandemic necessity of remote proceedings proved that virtual depositions could be equally effective while dramatically reducing costs and time investments.

Remote work acceptance extends beyond depositions to entire case management processes. Electronic medical record systems, secure file sharing platforms, and encrypted communication tools enable complete case analysis without ever meeting clients in person. This technological integration allows legal nurse consultants to serve national markets while maintaining flexible schedules and location independence.

Case management efficiency improved dramatically through digital transformation. Traditional paper-based record review required physical file storage, manual organization, and in-person meetings for case discussion. Modern electronic systems enable searchable databases, collaborative analysis platforms, and real-time communication with legal teams. A single legal nurse consultant can now manage multiple complex cases simultaneously using digital tools that would have required extensive support staff previously.

The shift also changed attorney expectations about consultant availability and responsiveness. Pre-pandemic communication often involved phone tag and delayed responses to urgent questions. Current practice expects near-immediate responses through multiple communication channels, but this increased connectivity comes with premium compensation for readily available expertise.

Technology adoption created new service opportunities for tech-savvy legal nurse consultants. **Electronic health record analysis** requires specialized skills in navigating different hospital systems, understanding data export formats, and identifying electronic documentation patterns that may not appear in printed records. Nurses who master these technical skills command premium rates for their enhanced capabilities.

Emerging Specializations: AI Litigation, Telehealth, Cybersecurity

The legal landscape continues expanding into areas that require specialized nursing expertise combined with emerging technology understanding. **Artificial intelligence in healthcare** creates new liability questions when diagnostic algorithms fail or treatment recommendations prove inappropriate. Legal nurse consultants who understand both clinical decision-making and AI system limitations become invaluable for cases involving these technologies.

Dr. Patricia Williams, a former informatics nurse, built her practice around AI-related healthcare litigation. When a major hospital's diagnostic AI system failed to identify early-stage cancer in multiple patients, her expertise in both clinical diagnostics and AI system design proved crucial to understanding liability issues. She explains: "Attorneys understand law, and technologists understand algorithms, but I understand how these systems interact with real patient care decisions."

Telehealth litigation represents another rapidly expanding specialty area. The pandemic's rapid telehealth adoption created numerous malpractice questions about remote care standards, technology failures, and diagnostic limitations. Legal nurse consultants with telehealth experience help attorneys understand when remote care decisions meet professional standards and when they constitute negligence.

Consider the case of Robert Kim, an emergency medicine nurse who transitioned to telehealth consultation during COVID-19. His dual experience in traditional emergency care and remote patient assessment made him perfect for analyzing telehealth malpractice claims. A recent case involved a patient who called a telehealth service with chest pain but died of myocardial infarction after being advised to take antacids. Robert's analysis showed the virtual provider's assessment failed to meet emergency care standards, despite technology limitations. His expert testimony helped secure a $3.2 million verdict.

Healthcare cybersecurity breaches create another emerging specialty requiring nursing expertise. When hospitals suffer data breaches or ransomware attacks, patient care often suffers delayed treatments, medication errors, and diagnostic delays. Legal nurse consultants who understand both clinical workflows and cybersecurity impacts help attorneys prove damages and establish liability.

The Colonial Pipeline ransomware attack in 2021 disrupted multiple hospital systems, leading to postponed surgeries and compromised patient monitoring. Legal nurse consultants helped attorneys understand how these disruptions affected patient outcomes and established causal relationships between cyber attacks and patient harm.

Pharmaceutical litigation continues expanding as new drugs reach market and long-term effects become apparent. The ongoing opioid litigation requires nurses who understand addiction medicine, pain management protocols, and pharmaceutical marketing practices. Similarly, emerging gene therapies and personalized medicine create liability questions requiring specialized nursing knowledge.

Self-Assessment: Are You LNC Material?

Legal nurse consulting attracts specific nursing personalities and skill sets, though success depends more on developed abilities than innate traits. **Analytical thinking** forms the foundation of effective legal nurse consulting. You must review complex medical records, identify patterns and inconsistencies, and draw logical conclusions about care quality and outcomes.

Ask yourself: Do you naturally question medical decisions and look for alternative explanations? When reviewing patient charts, do you notice inconsistencies between documentation and typical clinical practices? Can you explain complex medical concepts in simple terms that non-medical people understand? These analytical and communication skills predict success in legal nurse consulting better than any specific clinical background.

Attention to detail becomes crucial when analyzing medical records for legal purposes. A single missed medication, overlooked vital sign trend, or misinterpreted laboratory value can change case outcomes dramatically. Successful legal nurse consultants develop systematic review processes that ensure no critical information gets overlooked while maintaining efficiency in case analysis.

Communication skills prove equally important, but in different ways than traditional nursing requires. You'll need to write clear, concise reports that attorneys can use to build legal arguments. You'll explain medical concepts to juries composed of people without healthcare backgrounds. You'll collaborate with attorneys who think differently than healthcare professionals and have different priorities and timelines.

Independence and self-motivation separate successful legal nurse consultants from those who struggle. Unlike hospital nursing with constant supervision and structured schedules, legal consulting requires self-directed work, deadline management, and business development activities. You'll set your own schedule, manage multiple projects simultaneously, and take responsibility for marketing your services.

The most successful legal nurse consultants share certain characteristics: curiosity about how healthcare systems work, comfort with technology and electronic records, ability to see multiple perspectives on complex situations, and resilience when dealing with difficult or emotionally challenging cases. They also maintain objectivity when analyzing cases, regardless of personal feelings about patient outcomes or provider decisions.

Consider Lisa Park, a former medical-surgical nurse who initially struggled with legal consulting independence. Her hospital background emphasized teamwork and immediate supervisor availability for difficult decisions. Legal consulting required her to make independent judgments about complex cases without colleague input or supervisor guidance. She developed success through structured self-assessment protocols and regular professional development activities that built confidence in independent decision-making.

Previous legal experience is not required for legal nurse consulting success. Many successful practitioners had no legal background before beginning their consulting careers. However, willingness to learn legal concepts, understand court procedures, and adapt communication styles to legal audiences is essential for long-term success.

The self-assessment process should honestly evaluate your current situation and future goals. Are you seeking escape from bedside nursing's physical demands? Do you want intellectual challenges that traditional nursing cannot provide? Are you motivated by potential financial rewards or professional autonomy? Understanding your motivations helps determine readiness for the significant effort required to build a successful legal nurse consulting practice.

The legal nurse consulting revolution offers unprecedented opportunities for nurses ready to transform their careers and earning potential. The convergence of growing legal demand, technological advancement, and professional recognition creates ideal conditions for building successful consulting practices.

Your nursing background provides the foundation, but success requires commitment to developing new skills, understanding legal processes, and building professional relationships with attorneys. The investment in this career transformation pays dividends through increased income, professional satisfaction, and lifestyle flexibility that traditional nursing roles cannot match.

Key Takeaways from This Foundation

- Legal consulting represents a $20 billion industry with fewer than 5,000 specialized nurses serving over 1.3 million attorneys

- Geographic opportunities exist nationwide, with remote work eliminating traditional location barriers

- Income potential ranges from $150K-$300K+ annually for independent consultants, compared to $93K median RN salary

- Post-COVID technological changes permanently enabled remote legal nurse consulting practices

- Emerging specializations in AI litigation, telehealth, and cybersecurity offer premium compensation opportunities

- Success requires analytical thinking, attention to detail, communication skills, and self-motivation rather than specific clinical backgrounds

Chapter 2: Legal Nurse Consulting for Clinical Nurses

The gap between nursing school preparation and legal nurse consulting reality can feel overwhelming, particularly when existing resources assume legal knowledge you don't possess. You bring years of clinical experience, critical thinking skills, and patient care expertise—exactly what attorneys need—but the legal environment operates by different rules, timelines, and priorities than healthcare settings.

Understanding these differences while recognizing your existing strengths creates the foundation for successful transition. Legal nurse consulting doesn't require you to become an attorney or abandon your nursing identity. Instead, you'll apply your clinical expertise in new contexts that help attorneys understand medical complexities they cannot grasp independently.

What LNCs Actually Do Day-to-Day

Medical record analysis consumes the largest portion of most legal nurse consultants' time, but this analysis differs significantly from clinical chart review. Instead of looking for immediate patient care needs, you're identifying care standard deviations, missing documentation, and patterns that suggest negligence or appropriate care.

A typical medical record review begins with organizing records chronologically and by source (hospital, physician office, laboratory, imaging). You'll create timelines showing key events, treatments, and outcomes while noting gaps in documentation or care. This process might take 8-12 hours for a complex case involving multiple hospitalizations and providers.

Consider the case analysis completed by former cardiac nurse Michael Stevens. A 67-year-old patient died following routine cardiac catheterization, and the family alleged negligent post-procedure monitoring. Michael's analysis revealed the patient showed classic signs of cardiac tamponade—falling blood pressure, rising heart rate, and decreased urine output—for three hours before intervention. His report documented each vital sign abnormality and explained why competent nurses should have recognized the emergency. The attorney used Michael's timeline to show clear negligence patterns, resulting in a $1.8 million settlement.

Case consultation involves ongoing communication with attorneys about medical issues throughout litigation. You might receive calls asking about medication interactions, typical recovery timelines, or standard care protocols for specific conditions. These consultations typically last 15-30 minutes but require immediate availability and clear explanations of complex medical concepts.

Report writing transforms your analysis into documents attorneys can use for case strategy, settlement negotiations, or trial preparation. A typical case report includes chronological summary, care standard analysis, causation opinion, and damage assessment. These reports range from 5-20 pages depending on case complexity and might take 8-15 hours to complete properly.

Expert witness preparation represents the most challenging and highest-paid aspect of legal nurse consulting. You'll review case materials with attorneys, practice testimony techniques, and prepare for aggressive cross-examination by opposing counsel. This preparation might require 20-40 hours for complex cases but generates premium fees of $250-400 per hour plus appearance fees.

Deposition attendance allows you to observe expert witnesses, understand questioning techniques, and gain insights into legal strategies. Many legal nurse consultants attend depositions as observers before testifying themselves, learning how medical testimony fits into broader legal arguments.

The daily schedule varies dramatically based on case load and deadlines. Some days involve uninterrupted record review and analysis. Others include multiple attorney consultations, report writing, and case research. The flexibility appeals to many nurses, but it requires strong time management skills and ability to prioritize competing demands.

Employee vs Independent Contractor vs Expert Witness Roles

Insurance company employees represent the most traditional legal nurse consulting positions, offering steady income and comprehensive benefits while requiring less business development effort. These roles typically involve reviewing medical records for claim validity, identifying potential fraud, and recommending claim approvals or denials.

Jennifer Walsh worked as a claims review nurse for a major insurance company after 12 years in emergency nursing. Her daily responsibilities included reviewing emergency department records to determine if treatment met medical necessity criteria and identifying cases requiring additional investigation. The position offered $72,000 annually with full benefits, regular business hours, and no weekend or holiday work. Jennifer explains: "The transition felt natural because I was still applying my clinical knowledge, just in a different context."

Insurance positions typically require 2-5 years of clinical experience and prefer nurses with backgrounds in acute care, emergency medicine, or critical care. The work involves high-volume case review with emphasis on efficiency and consistency. Career advancement opportunities include senior review positions, training roles, and management positions within claims departments.

Law firm employees work directly for attorneys on litigation cases, combining medical record analysis with litigation support activities. These positions offer exposure to diverse case types and direct attorney interaction while providing stable employment structure.

Robert Chen transitioned from ICU nursing to a position with a personal injury law firm specializing in medical malpractice. His role includes reviewing potential cases for merit, preparing medical chronologies, and assisting with expert witness preparation. The firm paid $78,000 annually plus bonuses based on case outcomes. Robert's medical background helped attorneys understand complex ICU cases they previously struggled to evaluate properly.

Independent contractor arrangements offer maximum flexibility and earning potential while requiring significant business development and administrative responsibilities. You'll market your services, negotiate contracts, manage client relationships, and handle all business operations independently.

Dr. Sandra Kim, a former nurse practitioner, built an independent practice focusing on pharmaceutical litigation. Her expertise in pharmacology and patient management made her valuable for cases involving drug side effects and medication errors. Within three years, her practice generated $180,000 annually working approximately 30 hours per week. The independence allowed her to choose cases aligned with her expertise and interests while commanding premium rates for specialized knowledge.

Expert witness roles represent the highest compensation level but require extensive experience and exceptional communication skills. Expert witnesses provide opinions about care standards, causation, and damages while defending those opinions under aggressive cross-examination.

The transition from consultant to expert witness typically requires 3-5 years of legal nurse consulting experience plus additional training in testimony techniques. Expert witnesses must demonstrate credibility through education, experience, and previous testimony history. Compensation ranges from $250-400 per hour for preparation and testimony, with some experts earning $500+ per hour for highly specialized cases.

Myths vs Reality: Common Misconceptions Debunked

Myth: You need legal education to succeed as a legal nurse consultant. Reality: Your nursing education and clinical experience provide the foundation attorneys need most. Legal concepts can be learned through focused study and practical experience. Many successful legal nurse consultants never attended law school or completed legal education programs.

The legal industry values practical clinical knowledge over theoretical legal understanding. Attorneys need consultants who understand patient care realities, not legal theory. Your ability to identify care deviations, explain medical procedures, and predict patient outcomes matters more than knowing civil procedure rules or evidence standards.

Myth: Legal nurse consulting requires expensive certification programs. Reality: While certification can enhance credibility, many successful consultants build practices without formal certification. The industry-standard LNCC certification requires 2,000 hours of experience plus five years of nursing practice—a circular requirement that blocks entry for most newcomers.

Alternative credentials like CLNC certification cost less and require no experience prerequisites, but employer recognition varies. Many successful consultants build credibility through case results and attorney referrals rather than certification credentials. Focus on developing practical skills and building professional relationships rather than pursuing expensive certification programs immediately.

Myth: You must specialize in one clinical area. Reality: Generalist knowledge often proves more valuable than narrow specialization. Medical malpractice cases involve multiple clinical areas, and personal injury claims require understanding diverse medical conditions and treatments.

Mary Rodriguez, a former medical-surgical nurse, worried her generalist background wouldn't appeal to attorneys. Instead, her broad clinical experience helped her analyze complex cases involving multiple body systems and various medical specialties. Her ability to understand connections between different medical conditions and treatments made her valuable for cases requiring comprehensive analysis rather than narrow expertise.

Myth: Legal nurse consulting means abandoning patient care principles. Reality: Legal nurse consulting often improves patient care by identifying system failures and care deficiencies that led to patient harm. Your analysis helps prevent similar incidents while ensuring accountability for substandard care.

Successful legal nurse consultants maintain objectivity while honoring their nursing commitments to patient advocacy. When analysis reveals appropriate care, you'll support healthcare providers. When evidence shows negligence, you'll advocate for patients who suffered preventable harm. This balance maintains professional integrity while serving legal system needs.

Myth: The work is too emotionally difficult for caring nurses. Reality: While some cases involve tragic outcomes, the analytical nature of legal consulting provides emotional distance from immediate patient suffering. You're examining past events rather than providing direct patient care during crisis situations.

The emotional satisfaction of identifying care failures that led to preventable harm often outweighs the distress of reviewing tragic cases. Many legal nurse consultants find the work more emotionally sustainable than bedside nursing, which involves constant exposure to patient suffering and death.

Success Stories: Nurses Who Made the Transition

Patricia Thompson's transformation from burned-out ICU nurse to successful legal consultant illustrates the potential for career rejuvenation through legal nurse consulting. After 18 years in critical care, Patricia felt exhausted by constant patient deaths, understaffing, and administrative burdens that left little time for actual patient care.

Her introduction to legal nurse consulting came through jury duty in a medical malpractice case. Listening to expert testimony about critical care standards, Patricia realized she could explain the issues more clearly than the expensive expert witness. She began researching legal nurse consulting opportunities and completed a certification program within six months.

Patricia's first case involved ventilator management in a patient who developed pneumonia during prolonged mechanical ventilation. Her analysis revealed multiple care standard deviations: inadequate oral care, improper positioning, and delayed weaning attempts. The attorney had struggled to understand these technical issues until Patricia's report explained how each deviation contributed to the patient's infection and prolonged recovery.

The case generated $8,500 in fees over three weeks of part-time work. More importantly, the attorney referred Patricia to colleagues handling similar cases. Within one year, her legal consulting income exceeded her hospital salary, allowing her to leave bedside nursing permanently. Five years later, Patricia's practice generates over $200,000 annually while providing intellectual satisfaction and professional autonomy her hospital career never offered.

Dr. James Mitchell's transition from nurse practitioner to expert witness demonstrates how advanced practice experience translates into premium legal consulting opportunities. James practiced family medicine for 15 years in rural settings, gaining extensive experience with diverse medical conditions and limited resources typical of small-town healthcare.

His legal consulting career began when a local attorney asked for help understanding a case involving delayed diagnosis of diabetic ketoacidosis in the emergency department. James's analysis revealed that resource limitations didn't excuse the failure to recognize classic symptoms or order appropriate laboratory tests. His report helped secure a favorable settlement for the patient's family.

Word spread about James's analytical abilities and clear communication style. Attorneys began requesting his services for cases involving primary care issues, diagnostic delays, and rural healthcare standards. His unique combination of advanced practice experience and rural healthcare understanding made him valuable for cases other consultants couldn't properly evaluate.

James now commands $350 per hour for expert witness work, focusing on cases involving family practice, internal medicine, and rural healthcare issues. His testimony has influenced verdicts exceeding $10 million in total damages. The intellectual challenge and professional recognition far exceed what his clinical practice provided, while the income allows financial security he never achieved through patient care alone.

Lisa Park's gradual transition shows how legal nurse consulting can complement traditional nursing rather than replacing it immediately. Lisa continued working in medical-surgical nursing while building her consulting practice slowly over two years.

Her cautious approach began with small cases requiring minimal time investment. A slip-and-fall case needed someone to review emergency department records and explain injury patterns. The four-hour analysis earned $500—not significant money, but valuable experience in legal report writing and attorney communication.

As Lisa's skills developed and attorney relationships strengthened, case complexity and compensation increased. She began handling medical malpractice cases requiring extensive record analysis and expert opinions. The consulting work provided intellectual stimulation missing from routine hospital nursing while generating supplemental income.

After 18 months of part-time consulting, Lisa's legal work generated enough income to reduce her hospital schedule to part-time. This transition period allowed skill development and income replacement without the financial risk of immediate career change. She eventually left hospital nursing entirely when consulting income exceeded her full-time nursing salary.

Timeline Expectations: When Will You See Income?

Immediate income opportunities exist for nurses with specific skills or backgrounds attorneys need urgently. Emergency medicine nurses can often find consulting work within 30-60 days through personal injury attorneys handling accident cases. Critical care nurses may quickly locate opportunities with firms handling birth injury or surgical malpractice cases.

However, building a sustainable practice requires longer-term relationship development and skill refinement. Most successful legal nurse consultants report 6-12 months between initial training and regular income generation. This timeline includes completing education requirements, developing professional materials, networking with attorneys, and completing first cases that generate referrals.

The first six months typically involve significant effort with minimal income. You'll spend time learning legal processes, developing marketing materials, attending networking events, and completing initial cases at reduced rates to gain experience and references. Many new legal nurse consultants earn $2,000-5,000 during their first six months while investing 10-15 hours weekly in practice development.

Months 6-12 usually show accelerating income as attorney relationships develop and case complexity increases. Consultants often earn $8,000-15,000 during this period while establishing reputations for quality work and reliable service. Referrals from satisfied clients begin generating new opportunities without active marketing effort.

Year two and beyond typically achieve stable income levels for consultants who persist through initial challenges. Many part-time consultants earn $25,000-40,000 annually while maintaining other employment. Full-time practitioners often achieve $75,000-125,000 in annual revenue once practices mature.

The timeline varies significantly based on local market conditions, networking effectiveness, and case availability. Urban areas with multiple law firms and high litigation activity typically offer faster income development. Rural areas may require longer development periods but often provide less competition and stronger attorney relationships once established.

Factors that accelerate income development include previous legal experience, specialized clinical backgrounds, effective networking skills, and willingness to accept cases outside preferred comfort zones. Consultants who focus exclusively on high-paying expert witness work often struggle initially because this role requires extensive experience and credibility development.

Those willing to start with lower-paying analysis work, claims review, or basic consulting services typically achieve income goals faster while building skills needed for premium consulting roles later.

Investment Requirements and ROI Analysis

Initial investment requirements for legal nurse consulting remain modest compared to most business ventures, typically ranging from $2,000-8,000 depending on education choices and practice setup decisions. This investment includes education costs, professional materials development, technology purchases, and initial marketing expenses.

Education costs vary dramatically based on program selection. University-based certificate programs typically cost $3,000-8,000 and provide comprehensive theoretical foundation with academic credibility. Private certification programs range from $500-3,000 and focus on practical skills development. Self-study approaches using books and online resources may cost under $500 but require significant self-discipline and longer skill development timelines.

Technology investments include computer equipment, software licenses, and communication tools necessary for modern legal consulting practice. Essential technology includes reliable computer with large screen for document review, high-speed internet connection, scanner for document processing, and secure email system for confidential communications. These items typically cost $1,500-3,000 initially.

Professional software enhances efficiency and credibility but isn't required for initial practice development. Adobe Acrobat Pro ($200 annually) enables advanced document manipulation. Case management software ranges from $50-200 monthly depending on features and user requirements. Medical reference databases cost $100-500 annually but provide valuable resources for complex case analysis.

Marketing investments include professional website development, business cards, networking event attendance, and professional association memberships. Website development costs range from $500 for basic templates to $3,000 for custom professional design. Professional materials including business cards, letterhead, and marketing brochures typically cost $200-500 initially.

Professional association memberships provide networking opportunities and continuing education but require annual investments of $200-800 depending on organizations selected. The American Association of Legal Nurse Consultants charges $350 annually for full membership, while state nursing associations typically charge $100-200 annually.

Return on investment calculations show impressive potential for successful legal nurse consultants. A consultant earning $150,000 annually achieves 1,500-7,500% ROI on initial investments within the first year. Even modest success generating $30,000 annually provides 375-1,500% ROI depending on initial investment levels.

The calculation improves when comparing legal nurse consulting investments to traditional nursing education costs. Many nurses invested $40,000-100,000 in nursing education to achieve median salaries of $93,600. Legal nurse consulting education costing $2,000-8,000 can generate comparable or superior income levels with significantly lower educational investment.

Risk mitigation strategies include maintaining nursing employment during initial practice development, starting with part-time consulting to test market demand, and focusing on low-cost marketing approaches that generate attorney relationships without significant expenses.

The financial risk remains minimal because legal nurse consulting doesn't require inventory, physical office space, or employee hiring.

Most expenses are one-time investments in education and technology that retain value regardless of practice success levels.

Stepping Into Your Future

Legal nurse consulting represents more than career change—it's professional transformation that honors your nursing expertise while opening new opportunities for intellectual growth and financial success. The myths and misconceptions that discourage nurses from exploring this path often reflect outdated information or fear of the unknown rather than actual barriers to success.

Your clinical experience provides exactly what attorneys need most: practical understanding of patient care realities that no amount of legal education can provide. The investment required for this career transition remains modest, while the potential returns—both financial and professional—far exceed those available through traditional nursing advancement.

Essential Points for Your Journey

- Legal nurse consulting applies your clinical expertise in new contexts that help attorneys understand medical complexities

- Employment options range from stable insurance positions to independent practices with unlimited earning potential

- Success requires clinical knowledge and communication skills rather than legal education or expensive certification

- Realistic timelines show 6-12 months for regular income development, with sustainable practices achieved in 1-2 years

- Initial investments of $2,000-8,000 can generate returns of 375-7,500% within the first year of practice

- Risk remains minimal while maintaining nursing employment during transition periods

Chapter 3: Legal System Fundamentals for Nurses

The legal system operates by rules and procedures that seem foreign to healthcare professionals accustomed to clinical protocols and medical decision-making processes. Yet understanding these fundamental concepts doesn't require law school education—you need practical knowledge about how cases develop, progress through courts, and reach resolution.

Attorneys depend on your clinical expertise precisely because they lack medical knowledge, but they expect you to communicate using legal frameworks and understand how your analysis fits into broader case strategies. This chapter provides the essential legal foundation you need without overwhelming detail that obscures practical application.

Civil vs Criminal Law Basics

Civil law addresses disputes between private parties seeking financial compensation for harm or damages. Medical malpractice lawsuits, personal injury claims, and workers' compensation cases all fall under civil law jurisdiction. The goal is making injured parties "whole" through monetary awards rather than punishing wrongdoers.

Civil cases require proof by "preponderance of evidence"—meaning more likely than not that defendant actions caused plaintiff harm. This standard equals roughly 51% certainty that your analysis accurately identifies causation between medical care and patient outcomes. You don't need absolute certainty, just reasonable confidence based on available evidence.

Consider the case analyzed by former ER nurse David Martinez involving a delayed appendicitis diagnosis. The patient presented with abdominal pain but was discharged with gastroenteritis diagnosis. Twelve hours later, the appendix ruptured, requiring emergency surgery and prolonged hospitalization. David's analysis showed the initial symptoms were more consistent with appendicitis than gastroenteritis, and reasonable emergency medicine standards required additional testing before discharge. The preponderance of evidence supported the conclusion that delayed diagnosis caused the complications, leading to a $185,000 settlement.

Criminal law involves government prosecution of individuals who violated public laws and safety standards. Healthcare fraud, controlled substance diversion, and patient abuse cases fall under criminal jurisdiction. The goal is punishment through fines, imprisonment, or professional license suspension rather than victim compensation.

Criminal cases require proof "beyond reasonable doubt"—the highest legal standard requiring near-certainty about guilt. As a legal nurse consultant, you might analyze criminal cases involving healthcare providers accused of patient harm, but your role focuses on medical evidence analysis rather than guilt determination.

The practical difference affects how you approach case analysis and opinion formation. Civil cases allow qualified opinions acknowledging uncertainty while still identifying likely causation patterns. Criminal cases require more conservative analysis focusing on clear evidence of care standard violations without speculation about possible explanations.

Most legal nurse consultant work involves civil litigation, particularly medical malpractice and personal injury cases. Understanding this distinction helps you provide appropriate analysis depth and certainty levels that match legal requirements and attorney expectations.

How Medical Malpractice Cases Actually Work

Medical malpractice elements require proof of four specific components: duty, breach, causation, and damages. Each element must be established through evidence and expert testimony before successful case resolution. Your analysis typically addresses breach and causation elements where clinical expertise provides unique value.

Duty establishes the legal obligation between healthcare provider and patient. This element rarely requires extensive analysis because patient-provider relationships are usually well-documented through medical records, appointment schedules, and billing records. Hospital admission creates duty for all treating staff, while outpatient visits establish duty for specific providers involved in care decisions.

Breach identifies specific actions or omissions that violated accepted care standards. This element requires your clinical expertise to determine what competent healthcare providers would have done in similar circumstances. You'll compare actual care provided against professional standards established through literature review, guideline analysis, and peer practice patterns.

Former ICU nurse Margaret Wilson analyzed a case involving post-operative monitoring after cardiac surgery. The patient developed signs of internal bleeding—dropping blood pressure, increasing heart rate, and decreasing urine output—but nursing staff didn't notify surgeons for four hours. Margaret's analysis revealed that competent critical care nurses would have recognized these signs within 30 minutes and immediately contacted surgeons. The delay violated basic critical care standards and constituted clear breach of duty.

Causation connects care standard violations to specific patient harm. This element challenges many legal nurse consultants because medical causation involves complex interactions between multiple factors. You must distinguish between care failures that directly caused harm and those that were present but didn't contribute to negative outcomes.

The causation analysis requires understanding both factual causation ("but for" this error, would harm have occurred?) and proximate causation (was the harm a foreseeable result of the error?). Complex medical cases often involve multiple potential causes, requiring careful analysis to isolate contributions from care standard violations.

Damages quantify financial losses resulting from malpractice. These calculations typically involve economist experts rather than legal nurse consultants, but your analysis helps establish the severity and permanence of injuries caused by care failures. You might provide opinions about required future medical care, disability levels, or life expectancy changes resulting from malpractice.

The malpractice process typically begins with attorney case screening using medical record review to determine if expert analysis shows potential merit. You might provide initial case evaluation helping attorneys decide whether to accept clients and invest in expensive litigation processes.

Pre-litigation investigation involves comprehensive medical record review, literature research, and expert consultant identification. This phase might require 20-40 hours of analysis for complex cases involving multiple providers and extended treatment periods. Your analysis helps attorneys understand medical issues and develop case theories before filing lawsuits.

Discovery phase includes depositions, document production, and expert witness preparation. You might assist with deposition question development, expert witness selection, and case strategy refinement as medical evidence emerges through discovery process.

Trial preparation involves detailed expert witness coaching, visual aid development, and settlement negotiation support. Your clinical knowledge helps attorneys understand jury perspective on medical evidence and develop presentation strategies that communicate complex medical concepts effectively.

Personal Injury, Workers' Comp, and Products Liability Simplified

Personal injury cases arise from accidents, negligence, or intentional acts causing physical harm to individuals. Motor vehicle accidents, slip-and-fall incidents, and recreational activity injuries generate significant litigation requiring medical expertise to understand injury patterns, treatment appropriateness, and recovery prognosis.

These cases often involve emergency medicine evaluation, orthopedic treatment, and rehabilitation services. Your nursing background in trauma care, wound management, and patient recovery provides valuable insights into injury severity, treatment necessity, and long-term prognosis that attorneys need for case valuation and strategy development.

Physical therapist-turned-legal consultant Susan Chen analyzed a motorcycle accident case involving multiple trauma. The patient suffered fractured ribs, pneumothorax, and closed head injury requiring intensive care treatment and prolonged rehabilitation. Insurance companies disputed the necessity of extended physical therapy and ongoing neurological care. Susan's analysis demonstrated that the injury pattern required exactly the treatment provided, and premature therapy termination would likely result in permanent disability. Her report helped secure a $750,000 settlement covering projected lifetime care needs.

Workers' compensation cases involve job-related injuries or illnesses requiring medical treatment and disability compensation. These cases often challenge causation because many conditions develop gradually or involve pre-existing conditions aggravated by work activities. Your clinical knowledge helps determine if medical conditions reasonably relate to job responsibilities and work environment exposures.

Occupational health experience proves particularly valuable for workers' compensation analysis, but general medical knowledge often suffices for causation determination. You'll analyze injury mechanisms, treatment appropriateness, and work capacity limitations resulting from job-related medical conditions.

Products liability cases involve injuries caused by defective medical devices, pharmaceuticals, or consumer products. These cases require understanding product design, manufacturing processes, and failure mechanisms that caused patient harm. Your medical device experience, medication knowledge, and patient monitoring skills provide insights into how product failures affect patient safety.

The massive litigation surrounding defective hip implants illustrates products liability complexity. Thousands of patients suffered metallosis, implant loosening, and tissue damage from poorly designed devices. Legal nurse consultants with orthopedic experience helped attorneys understand normal vs. abnormal implant performance, symptom patterns indicating device failure, and treatment requirements for implant complications.

Pharmaceutical litigation represents a growing products liability category requiring specialized knowledge about drug mechanisms, side effect profiles, and clinical trial data. The opioid epidemic generated massive litigation examining pharmaceutical marketing practices, prescribing guidelines, and addiction potential disclosure.

Legal nurse consultants with pharmacology backgrounds help attorneys understand complex drug interactions, appropriate prescribing patterns, and failure to warn patients about known risks. These cases often involve thousands of plaintiffs with similar injury patterns requiring efficient analysis systems and standardized evaluation protocols.

Understanding Legal Teams and Where You Fit

Plaintiff attorneys represent injured individuals seeking compensation for harm caused by negligence or misconduct. These attorneys typically work on contingency fee arrangements, receiving payment only when cases resolve favorably. They need legal nurse consultants to identify winnable cases, understand medical complexities, and prepare compelling evidence presentations.

Plaintiff firms often maintain ongoing relationships with trusted legal nurse consultants who provide reliable analysis and testimony. Building these relationships requires demonstrating clinical competence, legal understanding, and communication skills that help attorneys present medical evidence effectively.

Defense attorneys represent healthcare providers, institutions, and insurance companies facing malpractice claims. These attorneys focus on disproving negligence allegations, minimizing damage assessments, and achieving favorable settlements or trial verdicts. They need consultants who can identify care standard compliance and alternative causation explanations.

Defense work often provides steadier income because insurance companies maintain regular case loads requiring ongoing consultant services. However, some nurses feel uncomfortable defending healthcare providers they believe provided substandard care. Successful defense consultants maintain objectivity while acknowledging that most healthcare providers strive to provide appropriate care under difficult circumstances.

Insurance companies employ or contract with legal nurse consultants for claims review, fraud investigation, and coverage determination. These positions typically offer stable employment with regular business hours and comprehensive benefits. The work involves high-volume case review with emphasis on efficiency and consistency.

Government agencies use legal nurse consultants for healthcare fraud investigation, regulatory compliance review, and policy development. The Centers for Medicare & Medicaid Services, state health departments, and attorney general offices employ nurses with legal expertise to analyze complex healthcare issues requiring both clinical and legal understanding.

Expert witness coordination represents a specialized role where experienced legal nurse consultants help attorneys identify, evaluate, and prepare expert witnesses for testimony. This work requires extensive knowledge of expert qualifications, testimony strategies, and courtroom procedures that develop through years of litigation experience.

Your position within legal teams depends on case requirements, attorney preferences, and your experience level. New consultants typically start with basic record analysis and case screening. Experienced consultants might coordinate entire case strategies and supervise other healthcare experts.

Communication protocols vary significantly between legal teams and healthcare settings. Legal communications often involve formal written reports, structured meeting agendas, and documented decision-making processes that differ from informal healthcare team discussions.

Attorneys expect timely responses to questions, detailed documentation of analysis methods, and clear explanations of clinical reasoning supporting your conclusions. They also need advance warning about potential problems with case theories or expert witness qualifications that might affect litigation strategies.

Legal Terminology That Matters to LNCs

Standard of care defines the level of competence expected from healthcare providers with similar training in similar circumstances. This concept forms the foundation of malpractice analysis because breach requires proving that care fell below accepted professional standards.

Standards derive from multiple sources: professional guidelines, hospital policies, peer practice patterns, and expert testimony about appropriate care. You'll often research literature and guidelines to establish care standards for specific clinical situations, then compare actual care provided against these established benchmarks.

Causation links specific actions or omissions to patient harm through medical and legal analysis. Medical causation requires understanding physiological mechanisms connecting care failures to patient injuries. Legal causation focuses on foreseeability and directness of connections between actions and outcomes.

Proximate cause limits liability to foreseeable consequences of negligent actions. A medication error causing allergic reaction represents proximate cause, while the same error leading to a car accident during medical transport might not qualify because the connection is too remote and unforeseeable.

Damages encompass all losses resulting from negligent care, including medical expenses, lost income, pain and suffering, and reduced life expectancy. Your analysis might address future medical needs, disability levels, and care requirements resulting from malpractice that help attorneys calculate appropriate damage awards.

Discovery refers to the pre-trial process where parties exchange information and evidence. You might assist with written discovery responses, document production, and deposition preparation as cases progress through litigation.

Depositions involve sworn testimony recorded by court reporters outside of trial settings. You might attend depositions as observer, consultant, or witness depending on your role in specific cases. Understanding deposition procedures helps you prepare effective testimony and assist attorneys with witness preparation.

Expert witness designation requires specific qualifications and imposes strict testimony rules about opinion scope and foundation. Experts must demonstrate relevant education, experience, and specialized knowledge that qualifies them to provide opinions beyond common knowledge of laypersons.

Affidavit represents sworn written statements used to support legal motions or establish facts without live testimony. You might prepare affidavits summarizing case analysis or providing expert opinions for summary judgment motions or settlement negotiations.

Settlement resolves cases through negotiated agreements without trial verdicts. Most cases settle before trial, often influenced by expert analysis showing case strengths and weaknesses. Your analysis helps attorneys evaluate settlement offers and negotiate appropriate resolutions.

Verdict represents jury or judge decisions after trial proceedings. Understanding verdict factors helps you prepare testimony and case presentations that effectively communicate medical evidence to legal decision-makers.

Court System Overview and Case Lifecycle

Federal courts handle cases involving federal laws, constitutional issues, or disputes between citizens of different states exceeding

$75,000 in damages. Medical device litigation, pharmaceutical cases, and major malpractice claims often proceed through federal court systems due to interstate commerce issues or federal regulatory involvement.

State courts handle most medical malpractice, personal injury, and local healthcare litigation. Each state maintains different procedural rules, evidence standards, and damage calculation methods that affect case strategy and analysis requirements.

Trial courts conduct initial case proceedings including discovery, motion practice, and trial proceedings. Most legal nurse consultant work occurs at trial court level where factual disputes require medical expertise for resolution.

Appellate courts review trial court decisions for legal errors but rarely reexamine factual determinations. Appeals typically focus on procedural issues, jury instruction problems, or evidence admission disputes rather than medical evidence analysis.

Case lifecycle typically spans 2-4 years from initial filing to final resolution, though complex cases might require longer periods. Understanding typical timelines helps you plan workload and manage client expectations about analysis deadlines and testimony scheduling.

Pre-litigation investigation might require 6-12 months of medical record review, expert consultation, and case development before lawsuit filing. This phase often determines case viability and strategy direction based on medical evidence strength.

Pleading stage involves formal legal document filing establishing case claims and defenses. Medical issues identified during pre-litigation investigation influence complaint language and discovery strategy development.

Discovery phase typically lasts 12-18 months involving extensive document production, deposition testimony, and expert witness preparation. Most legal nurse consultant work occurs during discovery as parties develop medical evidence and prepare case strategies.

Trial preparation requires intensive expert witness coaching, visual aid development, and testimony rehearsal during the 3-6 months preceding trial dates. Cases often settle during this phase as parties evaluate trial risks based on expert analysis and testimony preparation.

Trial proceedings might last days or weeks depending on case complexity and evidence volume. Your testimony might constitute a small portion of overall trial proceedings, but effective presentation often determines case outcomes.

Post-trial activities include appeal evaluation, judgment collection, and case closure activities that might require additional consultant services depending on verdict outcomes and post-trial motions.

Building Your Legal Foundation

Understanding legal system fundamentals provides the framework for effective legal nurse consulting practice. You don't need comprehensive legal education, but grasping these essential concepts enables clear communication with attorneys and appropriate analysis that serves legal case requirements.

The legal system values practical medical knowledge over theoretical legal understanding. Your clinical expertise remains your greatest asset, but communicating that expertise using legal frameworks and terminology enhances your effectiveness and professional credibility within legal environments.

Core Legal Concepts for Success

- Civil law seeks compensation through preponderance of evidence standards requiring 51% certainty in analysis conclusions

- Medical malpractice requires proving duty, breach, causation, and damages through clinical expertise and evidence analysis

- Personal injury, workers' compensation, and products liability cases apply medical knowledge to diverse legal contexts

- Legal teams include plaintiff attorneys, defense counsel, insurance companies, and government agencies with different priorities and needs

- Essential terminology includes standard of care, causation, damages, discovery, depositions, and expert witness requirements

- Court systems and case lifecycles span 2-4 years with most consultant work occurring during 12-18 month discovery phases

Chapter 4: Medical Record Analysis Mastery

Medical record analysis forms the cornerstone of legal nurse consulting—yet most nurses approach this task using clinical review habits that miss the legal significance hidden within documentation patterns. You'll discover that legal analysis requires a completely different mindset than patient care review, focusing on gaps, inconsistencies, and deviation patterns that attorneys need to build compelling cases.

The difference between clinical chart review and legal analysis mirrors the difference between treating a patient and solving a detective case. Clinical review seeks immediate care needs and treatment responses. Legal analysis searches for evidence of care failures, missed opportunities, and causal relationships that determine case outcomes and financial awards.

Systematic Review Protocols for Accuracy and Efficiency

The chronological foundation provides the most reliable starting point for comprehensive medical record analysis. You must organize all records by date and time, creating a timeline that reveals care patterns invisible in random chart review. This systematic approach prevents missing critical events and ensures accurate sequence understanding that attorneys need for case presentation.

Begin every analysis by collecting records from all sources—hospitals, physicians' offices, emergency departments, laboratories, imaging centers, and therapy providers. Missing even one source can create gaps that undermine your entire analysis. Create a master list documenting all record sources and page counts to verify completeness before beginning detailed review.

The three-pass system maximizes accuracy while maintaining efficiency in complex case analysis. The first pass involves organizing records chronologically and identifying key events without detailed analysis. This overview helps you understand the case scope and identify areas requiring focused attention.

During the second pass, analyze each record source separately, noting care decisions, treatment responses, and documentation quality. Create separate timelines for each provider showing their specific contributions to patient care. This step reveals communication breakdowns and coordination failures that often indicate substandard care.

The third pass integrates all provider timelines into a comprehensive case analysis, identifying patterns, gaps, and inconsistencies that suggest care standard violations. This systematic approach ensures no critical information gets overlooked while maintaining efficiency for time-sensitive attorney deadlines.

Consider the systematic analysis completed by former surgical nurse Rebecca Martinez on a post-operative infection case. The patient developed severe abdominal sepsis following routine gallbladder surgery, requiring multiple additional surgeries and prolonged hospitalization. Rebecca's three-pass analysis revealed the infection pattern:

First pass organization showed surgery on Monday, fever development Tuesday, antibiotic start Wednesday, and emergency surgery Friday. This timeline suggested possible care delays requiring detailed investigation.

Second pass analysis of nursing notes revealed the patient complained of severe abdominal pain Tuesday evening, but nursing documentation showed pain medication administration without physician notification. Laboratory records showed elevated white blood cell count Wednesday morning, but physician notes didn't address this abnormal finding until Thursday afternoon.

Third pass integration demonstrated a clear 48-hour delay in recognizing and treating post-operative complications. The systematic analysis provided attorneys with specific timeframes and documentation evidence showing care standard violations that directly contributed to patient harm. The case settled for $1.2 million based on Rebecca's detailed timeline analysis.

Documentation matrix systems help track multiple variables across extended timeframes in complex cases involving numerous providers and extended treatment periods. Create spreadsheets or databases tracking vital signs, medications, treatments, and patient responses across time to identify patterns invisible in narrative review.

This systematic approach proves especially valuable for medication error cases, where you must track multiple drugs, dosing changes, and patient responses over weeks or months. The matrix reveals dangerous patterns like dose escalation without monitoring or failure to recognize drug interaction warnings.

Identifying Care Standard Deviations and Red Flags

Nursing care standard analysis requires understanding both universal nursing principles and specialty-specific protocols that guide competent patient care. You'll compare actual nursing actions against established standards from professional organizations, hospital policies, and accepted practice guidelines.

Critical care monitoring standards provide clear benchmarks for patient assessment frequency, vital sign parameters, and intervention triggers. When ICU nurses fail to notify physicians about declining blood pressure, rising heart rate, or decreasing urine output—classic signs of shock—this represents clear care standard violation.

Red flag identification involves recognizing patterns that suggest systematic care failures rather than isolated mistakes. Multiple medication errors, repeated documentation gaps, or consistent monitoring failures indicate deeper problems than single incidents. These patterns strengthen legal cases by showing systematic negligence rather than unavoidable complications.

Former emergency nurse Patricia Chen analyzed a case involving delayed stroke recognition in a 72-year-old patient presenting with confusion and weakness. The patient waited four hours in the emergency department before receiving CT scan and stroke team evaluation, missing the critical window for clot-busting therapy.

Patricia's analysis revealed multiple red flags: triage notes documented one-sided weakness and speech difficulties but assigned low priority level; nursing assessments every four hours showed progressive neurological decline without physician notification; physician notes focused on psychiatric causes despite obvious neurological symptoms; CT scan ordered six hours after arrival despite clear stroke protocols requiring immediate imaging.

Each red flag represented individual care standard violations, but the pattern showed systematic failure to recognize and respond to stroke symptoms. The combination of nursing assessment failures, physician diagnostic errors, and protocol violations created a compelling negligence case. The delayed treatment resulted in permanent disability that early intervention would have prevented, leading to a $2.8 million verdict.

Medication administration analysis focuses on the five rights of medication safety: right patient, right drug, right dose, right route, and right time. Violations of these fundamental principles often indicate nursing negligence, especially when proper protocols could have prevented patient harm.

High-alert medications like insulin, anticoagulants, and cardiac drugs require special attention because errors with these substances frequently cause serious patient harm. Look for missing blood glucose checks before insulin, inadequate bleeding monitoring with anticoagulants, or dangerous drug combinations that competent nurses should recognize and question.

Communication breakdown identification reveals failures in the chain of patient safety that often contribute to adverse outcomes. Nurses who fail to report abnormal findings, physicians who don't respond to nursing concerns, and shift-change communication gaps all represent care standard violations with legal implications.

The case analyzed by former pediatric nurse Jennifer Williams illustrates communication breakdown consequences. A six-year-old patient developed respiratory distress following tonsillectomy, but nursing concerns about rapid breathing and agitation weren't communicated effectively to the surgical team.

Jennifer's analysis showed nursing documentation of respiratory rate climbing from 24 to 48 breaths per minute over two hours, with notation of "appears anxious" and "breathing fast." However, physician notification didn't occur until the child developed obvious distress requiring emergency airway management.

The communication failure represented clear nursing standard violation because pediatric post-operative monitoring requires immediate physician notification for respiratory changes. The delay in recognition and treatment caused preventable complications requiring additional surgery and prolonged recovery.

Causation Analysis: Linking Events to Injuries

Medical causation requires establishing direct connections between care failures and patient harm through physiological reasoning and timeline analysis. You must show that specific care standard violations directly caused or significantly contributed to adverse outcomes rather than representing unfortunate coincidences.

The "but for" causation test asks: Would this harm have occurred if the care standard violation had not happened? If proper care would have prevented or minimized the injury, then causation exists. However, pre-existing conditions, disease progression, and treatment complications can complicate causation analysis.

Proximate causation limits liability to foreseeable consequences of care failures. A medication error causing allergic reaction represents proximate causation, while the same error leading to depression from disfiguring rash might not qualify because the psychological harm was not a foreseeable consequence of the medication mistake.

Former cardiac care nurse Michael Rodriguez analyzed a case involving delayed recognition of heart attack symptoms in a 58-year-old woman presenting to the emergency department with chest discomfort and nausea. The patient was treated for gastroenteritis and discharged, only to suffer massive heart attack six hours later.

Michael's causation analysis showed the patient's symptoms—chest pressure, nausea, and diaphoresis—represented classic female heart attack presentation requiring immediate cardiac evaluation. The emergency department's failure to obtain EKG or cardiac enzymes represented clear care standard violation.

The causation connection required demonstrating that proper evaluation would have revealed the heart attack in progress, allowing immediate treatment that could have prevented the massive cardiac damage. Michael researched literature showing that women often present with atypical symptoms, and standard protocols require cardiac evaluation for any chest discomfort in patients over 50.

The timeline showed progressive cardiac damage over the six hours between discharge and return. Michael's analysis demonstrated that early recognition and treatment would have prevented 80% of the cardiac damage, providing strong causation evidence. The case resulted in a $1.5 million settlement based on the clear causation connection between care failure and patient harm.

Alternative causation investigation requires considering other possible explanations for patient outcomes that might reduce or eliminate provider liability. Pre-existing conditions, genetic factors, patient non-compliance, and disease progression can all contribute to adverse outcomes independent of care quality.

However, care standard violations remain negligent even when alternative factors contribute to patient harm. The key question becomes: Did the care failure significantly contribute to the adverse outcome? Partial causation still supports liability claims, though damage awards might be reduced based on contributing factors.

Missing Records Detection and Gap Analysis

Systematic gap identification reveals missing documentation that might hide care failures or important medical events. Hospitals and providers sometimes lose or destroy records, either accidentally or intentionally, creating evidentiary gaps that suggest important information is being concealed.

Standard medical record components include physician notes, nursing documentation, medication administration records, laboratory results, imaging reports, therapy notes, and discharge planning documents. Missing any of these components for significant time periods suggests potential record destruction or poor documentation practices.

Timeline gap analysis identifies periods where normal documentation patterns are interrupted or absent. For example, if nursing notes appear every four hours throughout a hospitalization but show a 12-hour gap during the period when complications developed, this missing documentation raises serious questions about care quality and record integrity.

Former orthopedic nurse Sarah Thompson analyzed a case involving surgical site infection following knee replacement surgery. The patient developed severe infection requiring multiple additional surgeries and eventual leg amputation. Sarah's gap analysis revealed critical missing documentation:

Operating room records showed routine procedure completion at 3:30 PM, but post-operative nursing notes didn't begin until 7:45 PM—a four-hour gap during the critical immediate recovery period. Medication administration records showed no entries for pain medication during this same period, despite routine post-operative pain management protocols.

Post-operative day two showed complete absence of wound assessment documentation, despite hospital policies requiring daily surgical site evaluation. The missing documentation corresponded exactly with the timeframe when infection symptoms would have first appeared.

Sarah's analysis suggested either grossly inadequate care during critical periods or intentional destruction of records documenting substandard care. The systematic gaps couldn't be explained by normal documentation variations and suggested concealment of negligent care that contributed to the devastating infection.

Electronic health record gaps present different challenges than traditional paper record missing pages. EHR systems track user access, document creation times, and editing history that can reveal record manipulation or deletion attempts. However, system failures, user errors, and technical problems can also create legitimate documentation gaps.

Understanding EHR audit trails helps identify suspicious record patterns versus technical problems. Multiple chart entries with identical timestamps, extensive editing of original notes, or unusual user access patterns might indicate record tampering rather than normal clinical documentation.

Electronic Health Record Navigation and Challenges

EHR system variations create significant challenges for legal nurse consultants who must analyze records from multiple hospitals and clinics using different electronic platforms. Epic, Cerner, Meditech, and other major systems organize information differently and present clinical data using varying formats and terminology.

Each EHR system uses different templates, flow sheets, and documentation structures that affect how clinical information appears in printed or electronic record production. Understanding these system differences helps identify missing information that might exist in the EHR but wasn't included in record production.

Data export limitations mean that printed EHR records often exclude important clinical information available in the electronic system. Alert systems, trending data, clinical decision support warnings, and communication tools might not appear in standard record production requests, creating artificial gaps in available evidence.

Former informatics nurse David Park analyzed a medication error case where printed records showed routine insulin administration but missed the critical information that the EHR system generated multiple drug interaction warnings that nurses dismissed without physician consultation.

David's analysis required requesting specific EHR screen shots showing alert systems, medication administration scanning records, and electronic communication between staff members. These electronic elements revealed that nurses received clear warnings about dangerous insulin dosing but failed to follow protocols requiring physician notification before override.

The EHR analysis showed systematic safety system bypassing that wouldn't have been apparent from standard printed records. The electronic evidence provided compelling proof of nursing negligence that led to patient hypoglycemia and permanent brain damage.

Timestamp analysis in EHR systems reveals documentation patterns that might indicate after-the-fact charting or other irregularities. When multiple detailed nursing assessments show identical timestamps during busy clinical periods, this suggests batch documentation rather than real-time patient evaluation.

Late documentation entries, especially those created after adverse events or incident reports, raise questions about accuracy and completeness. EHR systems track when notes are created versus when they claim to document patient care, revealing discrepancies between stated and actual documentation timing.

Pattern Recognition Techniques for Complex Cases

Trend identification involves analyzing clinical data patterns over time to recognize deteriorating patient conditions that should have prompted intervention. Vital sign trends, laboratory value changes, and medication response patterns often show clear warning signs that competent providers should recognize and address.

Blood pressure dropping from 140/90 to 100/60 over six hours represents a dangerous trend requiring immediate intervention, even if individual readings might seem acceptable. Pattern recognition helps identify when providers failed to recognize and respond to obvious clinical deterioration.

Communication pattern analysis reveals systematic failures in information sharing between healthcare team members. When nursing documentation shows consistent concerns about patient condition but physician notes don't acknowledge these issues, this pattern suggests communication breakdown that might have contributed to adverse outcomes.

Former case manager Linda Foster analyzed a complex case involving multiple provider failures leading to preventable patient death. A 45-year-old patient underwent routine hernia surgery but developed complications requiring multiple transfers between different hospital units and consulting specialists.

Linda's pattern analysis revealed systematic communication failures throughout the hospitalization: surgical team notes focused on wound healing while ignoring respiratory symptoms documented by nursing staff; internal medicine consultant recommended cardiac evaluation that was never completed; pharmacy alerts about drug interactions were acknowledged but not addressed.

The pattern showed fragmented care where each provider focused on narrow specialty concerns without considering overall patient condition. No single provider bore complete responsibility, but the systematic communication failures created a perfect storm of missed diagnoses and delayed treatments that ultimately caused preventable death.

Documentation quality patterns help identify periods of substandard care through analysis of record completeness, timeliness, and clinical appropriateness. High-quality documentation includes detailed assessments, clear care plans, and appropriate responses to patient changes. Poor documentation often correlates with poor patient care.

Sparse nursing notes, generic assessment findings, and missing critical documentation often indicate periods when care quality declined. These patterns become especially significant when they correspond with timeframes when complications developed or patient condition deteriorated.

Mastering the Evidence Trail

Medical record analysis mastery requires systematic approaches that reveal evidence hidden within clinical documentation patterns. Your nursing background provides the clinical knowledge to understand medical significance, but legal analysis demands detective skills that uncover care failures attorneys need to prove negligence.

The systematic protocols, gap identification techniques, and pattern recognition skills outlined here form the foundation for reliable analysis that stands up to expert scrutiny and courtroom challenges. Practice these methods consistently to develop the analytical expertise that separates successful legal nurse consultants from those who struggle with complex case challenges.

Essential Skills for Record Analysis Excellence

- Systematic three-pass review protocols ensure accuracy while maintaining efficiency in complex case analysis

- Care standard deviation identification requires understanding universal nursing principles and specialty-specific protocols

- Causation analysis links specific care failures to patient harm through physiological reasoning and timeline analysis

- Gap analysis reveals missing documentation that might hide care failures or suggest record destruction

- EHR navigation skills help identify information limitations in printed records and reveal electronic evidence

- Pattern recognition techniques identify systematic care failures and communication breakdowns across extended timeframes

Chapter 5: Professional Writing for Legal Audiences

Your clinical documentation skills provide a foundation for legal writing, but attorneys require different communication styles than healthcare colleagues. Legal writing demands precision, clarity, and persuasive organization that helps attorneys understand complex medical issues and build compelling case arguments.

The transition from nursing documentation to legal report writing challenges many consultants because medical and legal audiences have different priorities, knowledge levels, and decision-making processes. You'll need to adapt your communication style while maintaining clinical accuracy and professional credibility.

Attorney Communication Styles and Preferences

Legal communication patterns differ significantly from healthcare team interactions in structure, formality, and purpose. Attorneys think in terms of evidence, precedent, and argument development rather than patient care coordination and treatment planning. Your communications must align with these legal thinking patterns to be effective.

Attorneys prefer written communications that provide clear documentation of advice, analysis, and recommendations. Phone conversations should be followed by email summaries confirming key points and decisions. This documentation trail protects both parties and ensures important information doesn't get lost in busy legal practice environments.

Precision and specificity matter more to attorneys than general clinical impressions or intuitive judgments. Instead of writing "the patient appeared unstable," specify "blood pressure dropped from

130/80 to 95/60 over two hours, heart rate increased from 78 to 110, and urine output decreased from 50 ml/hour to 15 ml/hour."

This precision helps attorneys understand exactly what happened and why it matters legally. Vague statements like "poor nursing care" or "inappropriate treatment" provide no useful information for legal argument development. Specific care standard violations with clear explanations serve attorney needs much better.

Time-sensitive responsiveness reflects legal practice demands that operate under strict court deadlines and case development timelines. Attorneys often need immediate responses to urgent questions about medical issues affecting case strategy, settlement negotiations, or trial preparation.

Former emergency nurse Sandra Kim learned this lesson when an attorney called at 4 PM asking about medication interaction effects for a trial beginning the next morning. Sandra's detailed response helped the attorney prepare effective cross-examination questions that revealed opposing expert witness knowledge gaps. The attorney later explained that Sandra's quick, accurate response probably influenced the jury verdict in their favor.

Question anticipation shows legal thinking sophistication that attorneys appreciate in consultants. Instead of simply answering the specific question asked, consider related issues that might affect case strategy. This proactive analysis demonstrates understanding of legal needs beyond narrow clinical questions.

For example, if an attorney asks about blood loss calculation from surgical records, you might also address blood transfusion protocols, monitoring requirements, and symptoms that should have triggered earlier intervention. This broader analysis provides attorneys with complete information for case development rather than piecemeal responses to individual questions.

Medical Chronology Creation Step-by-Step

Chronological organization forms the backbone of effective legal case presentation because attorneys need to understand the sequence of medical events and care decisions that led to adverse outcomes. Your chronology becomes the roadmap that guides legal argument development and helps attorneys identify liability issues.

Begin chronology creation by establishing the relevant timeframe for analysis. Some cases require comprehensive review from initial symptoms through final resolution, while others focus on specific treatment periods when negligence allegedly occurred. Attorney guidance helps determine appropriate scope and detail level.

The three-column format provides optimal organization for legal chronology presentation: date/time, source, and event description. This structure allows attorneys to quickly locate specific information while maintaining clear understanding of event sequences and documentation sources.

Date/time entries should include precise timing when available, especially for critical events like medication administration, vital sign changes, or emergency interventions. Use 24-hour time format to avoid AM/PM confusion that can affect causation analysis and timeline accuracy.

Source identification helps attorneys understand evidence quality and potential credibility issues. Distinguish between physician notes, nursing documentation, laboratory reports, and patient/family statements because different sources carry different legal weight in case presentation.

For example, objective laboratory values carry more legal weight than subjective nursing assessments, while physician diagnostic decisions might be more legally significant than routine nursing care documentation. Understanding these distinctions helps you prioritize information appropriately.

Event description accuracy requires balancing completeness with readability for non-medical audiences. Include enough clinical detail for attorneys to understand medical significance while avoiding unnecessary medical jargon that obscures important points.

Consider this chronology excerpt from a medication error case analyzed by former ICU nurse Michael Rodriguez:

"10/15/24 0800 - Nursing assessment: Patient alert, oriented, blood glucose 180 mg/dL (normal 70-100). Regular insulin 10 units ordered per sliding scale protocol.

10/15/24 0815 - Medication administration record: Nurse Johnson administered 100 units regular insulin subcutaneously instead of ordered 10 units. Error noted in medication scanning system but override used without physician consultation.

10/15/24 0900 - Nursing note: Patient complained of feeling weak and dizzy. Blood glucose not rechecked despite symptoms consistent with hypoglycemia.

10/15/24 1000 - Laboratory result: Blood glucose 35 mg/dL (critically low). Patient found unresponsive, emergency response team called."

This chronology clearly shows the error sequence, missed intervention opportunities, and resulting patient harm in language attorneys can understand and present to juries effectively.

Case Summary Formats That Attorneys Love

Executive summary approach provides busy attorneys with essential case information in concise format that supports quick decision-making about case merit, settlement potential, and resource allocation. Lead with your conclusions, then provide supporting evidence and analysis.

The executive summary should answer three key questions within the first paragraph: Did negligence occur? Did negligence cause patient harm? What damages resulted from the negligence? This immediate clarity helps attorneys understand case value and development strategy.

Issue-focused organization structures complex cases around specific liability questions rather than chronological presentation. Group evidence by care standard violations, causation issues, and damage assessments to help attorneys prepare arguments and counter opposing claims effectively.

For example, organize a surgical malpractice case around pre-operative evaluation adequacy, intra-operative technique appropriateness, and post-operative monitoring compliance rather than simply listing events chronologically. This organization directly supports legal argument development.

Strength and weakness analysis demonstrates objective case evaluation that attorneys need for settlement negotiation and trial preparation. Acknowledge case weaknesses while explaining how they might be addressed through additional investigation or expert testimony.

Former surgical nurse Jennifer Washington analyzed a case involving post-operative bleeding complications following gallbladder surgery. Her summary identified case strengths (clear delay in recognizing bleeding, standard protocol violations, preventable complications) and weaknesses (patient obesity complicating surgery, previous surgical history, pre-existing bleeding disorder).

Jennifer's balanced analysis helped attorneys understand realistic case expectations and develop strategies for addressing weaknesses through expert testimony about obesity management and bleeding disorder protocols in surgical patients. The honest evaluation led to successful settlement negotiations based on realistic case valuation.

Visual presentation techniques help attorneys understand complex medical information through charts, timelines, and diagrams that supplement written analysis. Many attorneys learn better through visual presentation than dense text descriptions of medical events.

Consider creating timeline graphics showing care failures, flowcharts illustrating decision-making processes, or anatomical diagrams explaining injury mechanisms. These visual aids become powerful trial presentation tools that help juries understand complex medical issues.

Expert Opinions: When and How to Provide Them

Opinion scope limitations require understanding the difference between factual analysis and expert opinions that require special qualifications and legal foundation. You can always describe what medical records show and explain standard care protocols, but expert opinions about care standard violations require proper credentialing and case-specific foundation.

Factual statements describe what happened: "The nurse administered 100 units of insulin instead of the ordered 10 units." Expert opinions interpret significance: "This medication error represents a clear violation of safe medication administration practices." Know the distinction and stay within appropriate boundaries.

Qualification establishment for expert opinion testimony requires demonstrating relevant education, experience, and specialized knowledge that qualifies you to provide opinions beyond common knowledge. Your nursing background provides foundation, but specific case expertise requires additional credentials.

For medication error cases, your ICU experience with high-alert medications provides relevant background. For surgical cases, your operating room or post-operative experience becomes important.

Match your background to case requirements and acknowledge limitations honestly.

Opinion formation methodology requires systematic analysis based on established care standards, professional guidelines, and peer practice patterns rather than personal preferences or institutional practices. Document your research process and cite authoritative sources supporting your conclusions.

Begin opinion formation by researching applicable care standards from professional organizations, hospital accreditation requirements, and published clinical guidelines. Compare actual care provided against these established standards to identify violations objectively.

Language precision in expert opinions affects legal admissibility and persuasive impact. Use definitive language for clear violations ("This care fell below accepted standards") and qualified language for borderline cases ("This care appears to fall below accepted standards").

Avoid absolute statements unless evidence clearly supports certainty. Phrases like "in my opinion," "based on my experience," and "according to established standards" help establish appropriate foundation for expert opinions while acknowledging inherent limitations.

Former pediatric nurse Patricia Chen provided expert opinions in a case involving delayed recognition of meningitis in a six-year-old patient. Her opinion clearly stated: "Based on my 15 years of pediatric nursing experience and review of current pediatric assessment guidelines, the nursing staff's failure to recognize and report classic signs of meningitis—fever, neck stiffness, and altered mental status—fell below accepted pediatric nursing standards."

Patricia's opinion provided clear legal foundation by citing her relevant experience, referencing established guidelines, and using definitive language about the care standard violation. The opinion helped attorneys secure a favorable settlement based on clear expert analysis.

Avoiding Common Writing Mistakes That Lose Clients

Medical jargon overuse creates communication barriers that prevent attorneys from understanding your analysis and presenting medical evidence effectively to juries. Write for intelligent lay audiences rather than medical colleagues, explaining technical terms and concepts clearly.

Instead of writing "The patient developed ARDS secondary to sepsis with resultant hypoxemia requiring mechanical ventilation," explain "The patient developed severe lung inflammation caused by infection, resulting in dangerous oxygen levels that required breathing machine support."

Bias appearance undermines credibility when your writing suggests predetermined conclusions rather than objective analysis. Attorneys need balanced case evaluation that acknowledges strengths and weaknesses rather than advocacy pieces supporting only one perspective.

Avoid inflammatory language like "shocking negligence" or "inexcusable care failures" that suggests emotional rather than professional analysis. Present evidence objectively and let attorneys develop persuasive arguments based on your factual analysis.

Speculation beyond evidence weakens legal arguments when your analysis goes beyond what medical records actually document. Distinguish between what you can prove from available evidence versus what might have happened with additional information.

Use precise language that matches evidence certainty: "The records show..." for documented facts, "The evidence suggests..." for reasonable inferences, and "It's possible that..." for speculation beyond available evidence. This precision helps attorneys understand argument strength and potential challenges.

Organizational confusion frustrates attorneys when reports lack clear structure and logical flow between related concepts. Use headings, numbered sections, and topic sentences that guide readers through complex medical analysis efficiently.

Structure reports using legal thinking patterns: state conclusions first, then provide supporting evidence and analysis. This "bottom line up front" approach serves attorney needs better than medical case presentation formats that build toward diagnostic conclusions.

Templates and Examples for Immediate Use

Case analysis report template provides consistent structure for medical record review and opinion development that attorneys find helpful and professional. Standardize your reports using proven formats that cover essential elements systematically.

Header Section:

- Case identification (plaintiff name, case number)
- Date of analysis completion
- Consultant qualifications summary
- Records reviewed (sources and page counts)

Executive Summary (1-2 paragraphs):

- Key findings and conclusions
- Care standard violations identified
- Causation analysis results
- Damage assessment overview

Factual Background:

- Relevant medical history
- Treatment timeline
- Key healthcare providers
- Outcome summary

Analysis Sections:

- Care standard review
- Violation identification
- Causation analysis
- Alternative explanations considered

Conclusions and Opinions:

- Summary of findings
- Expert opinions (if qualified)
- Limitations and uncertainties
- Additional investigation recommendations

Medical chronology template provides attorneys with essential timeline information in accessible format that supports case development and presentation preparation.

Use spreadsheet format with columns for:

- Date/Time
- Source (physician note, nursing record, lab result)
- Event Description
- Clinical Significance
- Care Standard Implications

Email communication template ensures professional correspondence that documents important discussions and decisions while maintaining appropriate tone and content for attorney audiences.

Subject line: Case name - Specific topic Greeting: Professional but warm Purpose statement: Clear reason for communication Content: Organized bullet points or numbered items Action items: Specific next steps or decisions needed Closing: Professional sign-off with contact information

These templates provide starting points for developing your own communication styles and report formats that serve attorney needs while reflecting your professional standards and clinical expertise.

Writing Your Way to Success

Professional writing skills separate successful legal nurse consultants from those who struggle to build sustainable practices. Attorneys value consultants who communicate clearly, organize information effectively, and present medical analysis in formats that support legal argument development and case presentation.

Your clinical knowledge provides the foundation, but legal writing skills determine how effectively you can share that knowledge with attorney clients. Practice these communication techniques consistently to develop the professional writing expertise that generates client satisfaction and referral opportunities.

Core Writing Principles for Legal Success

- Attorney communication requires precision, documentation, and responsiveness that differs from healthcare team interactions

- Medical chronologies organize complex information using three-column format showing date/time, source, and event descriptions

- Case summaries lead with conclusions and organize evidence around liability issues rather than chronological presentation

- Expert opinions require proper qualification and careful language that distinguishes facts from professional interpretations

- Common writing mistakes include medical jargon overuse, bias appearance, speculation beyond evidence, and organizational confusion

- Professional templates ensure consistent quality and attorney-friendly formats for reports, chronologies, and communications

Chapter 6: Technology Tools for Modern LNC Practice

Technology transforms legal nurse consulting from paper-intensive manual processes into efficient digital practices that serve clients nationwide while reducing overhead costs and increasing analytical capabilities. You'll discover that mastering these tools separates successful modern consultants from those struggling with outdated methods that limit practice growth and client satisfaction.

The technological transformation accelerated dramatically during the COVID-19 pandemic, making remote legal nurse consulting not just possible but preferred by many attorneys. Digital tools now enable comprehensive case analysis, secure client communication, and professional presentation capabilities that were impossible just a few years ago.

Essential Software Suite: Adobe, CaseMap, MasterFile

Adobe Acrobat Pro serves as the foundation for digital document management in legal nurse consulting practice. This software enables advanced PDF manipulation, annotation, and organization capabilities essential for working with electronic medical records and creating professional deliverables for attorney clients.

Basic PDF viewing software cannot handle the complex document manipulation required for legal case analysis. Adobe Acrobat Pro allows document merging, page reordering, annotation layers, and advanced search capabilities across multiple large PDF files containing thousands of pages of medical records.

Document organization features include bookmark creation, page labeling, and section dividers that help attorneys navigate complex medical record sets efficiently. You can create clickable table of contents, insert divider pages between different record sources, and add descriptive headers that make document navigation intuitive for legal teams.

The annotation tools enable collaborative review processes with attorney clients. Highlight important passages, add comment bubbles explaining medical significance, and create sticky note annotations that provide additional context without altering original documents. These annotations can be saved separately or integrated into final documents based on client preferences.

Security and redaction capabilities protect patient privacy while enabling legal case analysis. Adobe Acrobat Pro includes redaction tools that permanently remove confidential information from documents, ensuring HIPAA compliance while preserving case-relevant medical information for legal review.

Former ICU nurse Sarah Martinez used Adobe Acrobat Pro to analyze a complex cardiac surgery case involving over 3,000 pages of records from six different hospitals. She created a master PDF with bookmarks for each hospitalization, annotated key cardiac monitoring entries, and redacted patient identifiers throughout. The organized document set allowed attorneys to quickly locate relevant information during depositions and trial preparation, contributing to a successful case outcome.

CaseMap software provides legal case management capabilities specifically designed for litigation support and evidence organization. This LexisNexis product helps legal professionals organize facts, people, issues, and evidence in structured databases that support case analysis and presentation development.

The software enables chronology creation, fact organization, and relationship mapping between case elements that traditional spreadsheets cannot handle effectively. You can link medical events to specific healthcare providers, connect care standard violations to patient outcomes, and track evidence sources throughout complex litigation processes.

Issue-based organization allows systematic analysis of legal questions through medical evidence review. Create separate issue categories for different liability theories—medication errors, monitoring failures, communication breakdowns—and link relevant facts and evidence to each issue category for efficient case development.

The relationship mapping features help visualize complex cases involving multiple providers, facilities, and time periods. CaseMap can generate timeline graphics, relationship charts, and issue summaries that serve as powerful litigation support tools for attorney clients.

MasterFile software specializes in legal nurse consulting workflows with features designed specifically for medical record analysis and case management. This software includes medical terminology databases, care standard references, and report templates tailored to legal nurse consulting needs.

The integrated medical references help verify care standards, medication information, and clinical protocols during case analysis. Built-in medical dictionaries, drug interaction databases, and clinical guideline references provide quick access to authoritative information needed for expert analysis.

Case tracking capabilities monitor multiple cases simultaneously with deadline alerts, task management, and progress tracking features designed for independent legal nurse consulting practices. The software integrates time tracking, billing, and client communication tools into unified case management systems.

Template libraries include standard report formats, chronology layouts, and correspondence templates that ensure consistent professional presentation across all client deliverables. Customizable templates allow adaptation to specific attorney preferences while maintaining professional standards.

AI-Powered Document Analysis Tools

Artificial intelligence applications in legal nurse consulting focus on pattern recognition, document classification, and preliminary analysis that enhances human expertise rather than replacing clinical judgment. These tools process large document volumes quickly while identifying potential issues that require detailed human analysis.

Current AI tools excel at organizing documents, extracting key data points, and identifying potential inconsistencies across large record sets. However, clinical judgment, care standard analysis, and expert opinion formation still require human expertise that AI cannot replicate effectively.

Document classification systems use machine learning to categorize medical records by type, date, and source automatically. These systems can separate physician notes from nursing documentation, organize laboratory results chronologically, and identify imaging reports within large document collections.

The time savings prove significant for cases involving extensive medical records from multiple sources. AI classification systems can process 1,000-page record sets in minutes, providing organized document collections that would require hours of manual sorting.

Text extraction and data mining capabilities identify specific medical terminology, medication names, and clinical findings across large document volumes. Advanced systems can locate all references to specific medications, track vital sign trends, and identify documentation gaps automatically.

Former emergency nurse David Park used AI-powered analysis tools for a medication error case involving insulin overdose. The AI system identified every reference to insulin throughout 500 pages of medical records, extracted all blood glucose values, and flagged timeline gaps in glucose monitoring. This automated analysis provided David with organized data that accelerated his detailed case analysis by several days.

Pattern recognition algorithms identify potential care standard violations by comparing documented care against established protocols and typical practice patterns. These systems can flag unusual medication dosing, abnormal vital sign responses, and documentation inconsistencies that warrant detailed investigation.

However, pattern recognition requires human verification because AI systems cannot distinguish between appropriate care variations and actual standard violations. The technology serves as analytical assistance rather than diagnostic replacement for clinical expertise.

Predictive analytics capabilities help identify cases with high litigation potential by analyzing multiple factors associated with successful malpractice claims. These systems consider injury severity, care standard deviations, and outcome preventability to help attorneys prioritize case investment decisions.

Legal nurse consultants can use predictive analytics to provide preliminary case screening that helps attorneys make informed decisions about case acceptance and resource allocation. However, final case merit determination still requires detailed human analysis and expert judgment.

Mobile Productivity Apps for Remote Work

Secure communication platforms enable confidential client interaction through encrypted messaging, voice calls, and video conferencing that meet HIPAA compliance requirements for protected health information discussion. Popular platforms include Signal, ProtonMail, and specialized legal communication tools.

Mobile apps allow immediate response to urgent attorney questions about case issues, depositions, or trial preparation needs. Quick consultation capabilities provide competitive advantages in legal markets where responsive expert support influences case outcomes and client satisfaction.

Cloud-based document access through secure platforms like Box, SharePoint, or specialized legal cloud services enables case analysis from any location with internet connectivity. Mobile document viewers allow preliminary review and note-taking even when comprehensive analysis requires desktop computer capabilities.

The ability to review case documents during travel, court appearances, or client meetings provides flexibility that enhances client service while maximizing productive time utilization. Mobile access becomes essential for consultants serving clients in multiple geographic markets.

Time tracking and billing applications designed for professional service providers help track case hours, calculate billing amounts, and generate client invoices directly from mobile devices. Popular options include Toggl, Harvest, and specialized legal billing software with mobile capabilities.

Accurate time tracking proves crucial for independent legal nurse consultants who bill hourly for case analysis, consultation services, and expert witness preparation. Mobile tracking ensures accurate recording of all billable activities regardless of location or work environment.

Voice-to-text capabilities enable dictation of case notes, preliminary observations, and follow-up reminders using smartphone voice recognition technology. Advanced systems can transcribe medical terminology accurately and integrate with case management software for seamless workflow integration.

Former pediatric nurse Jennifer Williams uses mobile dictation to record initial case impressions immediately after reviewing medical records. She dictates key findings, potential issues, and follow-up research needs while information remains fresh, then uses transcriptions to guide detailed written analysis later.

Reference applications provide instant access to medical information, drug databases, and clinical guidelines needed for case analysis. Popular medical reference apps include Epocrates, Lexicomp, and UpToDate mobile versions that offer offline access to essential clinical information.

Quick reference access proves valuable during client consultations, deposition attendance, and case discussions when immediate medical information retrieval enhances credibility and responsiveness to attorney questions.

HIPAA-Compliant Systems and Security Requirements

Protected health information regulations require specific security measures for any systems used to store, transmit, or process patient medical records during legal nurse consulting activities. HIPAA compliance extends beyond healthcare settings to include legal consultants handling medical information.

Business associate agreements with attorney clients establish mutual responsibilities for PHI protection and outline specific security requirements for consultant technology systems. These agreements typically require encryption, access controls, and audit trail capabilities for all PHI handling systems.

Encryption requirements mandate that patient information remain encrypted both during transmission and while stored on computer systems or cloud platforms. Advanced Encryption Standard (AES) 256-bit encryption represents current best practice for PHI protection in legal consulting environments.

Email systems must use end-to-end encryption when transmitting medical records or case discussions containing patient identifiers. Standard commercial email services like Gmail or Yahoo Mail do not meet HIPAA encryption requirements without additional security measures.

Access control systems limit medical record access to authorized personnel and maintain detailed logs of all system access attempts and file viewing activities. These controls include password protection, multi-factor authentication, and automatic logout features for unattended systems.

Cloud storage platforms must offer granular access controls that allow sharing specific documents with authorized attorney staff while preventing unauthorized access by other cloud users. Popular HIPAA-compliant cloud services include Box for Business, Microsoft 365 Government, and specialized legal cloud platforms.

Audit trail capabilities track all interactions with protected health information, including document access, modification attempts, and sharing activities. These logs provide evidence of appropriate PHI handling and help identify potential security breaches quickly.

The audit trails become especially important during litigation when opposing counsel might question medical record handling procedures or attempt to exclude evidence based on security concerns. Detailed logs demonstrate proper PHI protection throughout case analysis processes.

Incident response procedures establish protocols for responding to potential HIPAA violations, security breaches, or unauthorized PHI access attempts. These procedures include immediate containment measures, client notification requirements, and regulatory reporting obligations.

Legal nurse consultants must understand their obligations under business associate agreements and maintain incident response capabilities appropriate for their practice scope and technology utilization. Regular security training and system updates help prevent incidents that could compromise client relationships and professional reputation.

Virtual Deposition Platforms and Best Practices

Remote deposition technology evolved rapidly during the COVID-19 pandemic, transforming from emergency measures into preferred practice methods for many legal proceedings. Virtual depositions offer cost savings, scheduling flexibility, and geographic reach advantages that benefit both attorneys and expert witnesses.

Popular platforms include Zoom for Government, Microsoft Teams Government, and specialized legal platforms like Stenograph LiveDeposition and U.S. Legal Support RemoteDepo that offer enhanced security and legal-specific features designed for litigation support.

Technical setup requirements include high-quality camera and microphone equipment, reliable internet connectivity, and backup systems for technology failures during critical proceedings. Professional appearance and audio quality significantly impact witness credibility and testimony effectiveness.

Lighting setup affects visual presentation quality significantly. Position primary light sources in front of your face rather than behind to avoid backlighting that makes facial expressions difficult to see. Professional-quality webcams provide better image clarity than built-in laptop cameras for important depositions.

Professional presentation techniques adapt traditional deposition skills to virtual environments where body language, document handling, and attorney interaction occur through technology interfaces. Maintain eye contact with the camera rather than the screen to create appropriate visual connection with questioning attorneys.

Document review during virtual depositions requires additional preparation because traditional paper shuffling and physical document marking become more complex through screen sharing and digital annotation systems. Organize electronic documents with clear labeling and bookmark systems for efficient navigation during testimony.

Security considerations for virtual depositions include encrypted transmission, controlled access, and recording restrictions that protect confidential case information and attorney work product. Verify platform security features before participating in depositions involving sensitive medical information or trade secrets.

Former cardiac nurse Michael Rodriguez participated in a virtual deposition regarding post-operative monitoring standards in cardiac surgery cases. His careful technical preparation—professional lighting, high-quality audio, organized electronic documents— contributed to effective testimony that helped attorneys secure favorable case resolution. The virtual format allowed participation without expensive travel while maintaining professional presentation standards.

Backup contingency planning addresses potential technology failures that could disrupt important legal proceedings. Maintain alternative communication methods, backup internet connections, and secondary device options for critical deposition participation.

The planning should include primary platform testing, audio/video quality verification, and document access confirmation well before scheduled deposition times. Technology rehearsals with attorney clients help identify potential issues and develop solutions before actual proceedings.

Business Management Technology Integration

Client relationship management systems track attorney contacts, case progress, and communication history through specialized CRM platforms designed for professional service providers. These systems help maintain client relationships and identify referral opportunities systematically.

Legal-specific CRM platforms like Lexicata, Lawmatics, or general business systems like Salesforce provide contact management, communication tracking, and business development tools that support practice growth and client retention efforts.

Financial management integration connects time tracking, billing, and accounting systems to streamline practice administration and ensure accurate client invoicing. Popular combinations include QuickBooks Online with specialized time tracking apps that sync billing data automatically.

The integration eliminates duplicate data entry while providing detailed financial reporting that supports business decision-making and tax preparation. Automated systems reduce administrative overhead while improving billing accuracy and client satisfaction.

Project management platforms help coordinate multiple cases, deadlines, and deliverables through systems like Asana, Monday.com, or specialized legal project management tools. These platforms provide task tracking, deadline alerts, and progress monitoring for complex case analysis projects.

The systems prove especially valuable for consultants managing multiple attorney clients with different case timelines, reporting requirements, and communication preferences. Centralized project tracking prevents missed deadlines and ensures consistent service quality across all client relationships.

Marketing automation systems help independent legal nurse consultants maintain professional visibility through email marketing, social media management, and content distribution platforms. These systems enable consistent marketing efforts without significant time investment.

LinkedIn automation tools, email newsletter platforms, and content scheduling systems help maintain professional relationships and attract new clients through systematic marketing activities. However, automation must comply with professional ethics requirements for healthcare consultants and maintain authentic professional communication.

Data backup and recovery systems protect against catastrophic data loss that could destroy years of case analysis work and client communications. Cloud-based backup solutions provide automatic protection with geographic redundancy and disaster recovery capabilities.

The systems should include both real-time synchronization for active cases and periodic full backups of complete system data. Regular backup testing ensures recovery capabilities work properly when needed for actual system failures or security incidents.

Technological Transformation Success

Technology mastery separates modern legal nurse consultants from those struggling with outdated manual processes that limit practice efficiency and growth potential. The tools and systems outlined here provide the foundation for building scalable practices that serve clients effectively while maintaining professional standards and security requirements.

Your clinical expertise remains the core value proposition, but technological capabilities determine how effectively you can deliver that expertise to attorney clients seeking efficient, responsive, and professional consulting services. Invest in learning these systems to build sustainable competitive advantages in evolving legal markets.

Technology Integration Essentials for Practice Excellence

- Adobe Acrobat Pro, CaseMap, and MasterFile provide essential document management and case analysis capabilities for professional practice

- AI-powered tools enhance document processing efficiency while human expertise remains essential for clinical judgment and analysis

- Mobile apps enable responsive client service and flexible work arrangements that improve satisfaction and competitive positioning

- HIPAA-compliant systems protect patient privacy while meeting business associate agreement requirements for legal consulting

- Virtual deposition platforms require technical preparation and professional presentation skills adapted to remote environments

- Business management integration streamlines practice administration while supporting growth and client relationship development

Chapter 7: Beyond Medical Malpractice - Expanding Your Practice

Legal nurse consulting extends far beyond traditional medical malpractice cases into specialized practice areas that offer premium compensation and reduced competition. You'll discover that attorneys handling products liability, environmental health, workers' compensation, criminal defense, elder care, and family law cases desperately need medical expertise—yet most legal nurse consultants never explore these lucrative opportunities.

These diverse practice areas allow you to apply your nursing knowledge in contexts that traditional healthcare settings never provided while serving attorney clients who appreciate your clinical perspective on complex legal questions. Each specialty requires different analytical approaches but builds on the same foundation of medical knowledge that you already possess.

Products Liability and Medical Device Litigation

Medical device failures create massive litigation opportunities requiring nurses who understand both clinical applications and failure mechanisms that cause patient harm. Hip implants, cardiac devices, surgical instruments, and monitoring equipment generate thousands of lawsuits annually when design defects or manufacturing problems cause injuries.

The massive litigation surrounding defective hip implants illustrates the scope and complexity of medical device cases. Metal-on-metal hip replacements caused metallosis, tissue death, and implant failure in thousands of patients worldwide. Attorneys needed medical experts who understood normal hip function, implant design principles, and symptom patterns indicating device failure.

Case analysis requirements for device litigation focus on understanding normal device function, identifying failure mechanisms, and connecting device problems to specific patient injuries. You'll review medical literature, manufacturer documentation, and FDA safety communications to establish how devices should perform versus actual patient outcomes.

Former orthopedic nurse Sandra Martinez built her practice around hip implant litigation after witnessing multiple device failures during her hospital career. Her clinical experience with post-operative hip replacement patients provided unique insights into normal recovery patterns versus device-related complications.

Sandra's analysis of a 62-year-old patient who received a metal-on-metal hip implant revealed the progression from successful initial surgery to devastating device failure. The patient's symptoms—increasing hip pain, metallic taste, and muscle weakness—developed two years post-surgery and matched published reports of metallosis from metal wear debris.

Her medical record review showed physicians initially dismissed the patient's complaints as normal aging or arthritis progression. However, Sandra's analysis demonstrated that the symptom pattern, timing, and laboratory findings (elevated metal ion levels) clearly indicated device failure requiring immediate revision surgery.

The case required Sandra to research hip implant design, metallurgy principles, and toxicology data showing how metal debris damages surrounding tissue. Her analysis helped attorneys understand the technical aspects of device failure while maintaining focus on patient impact and preventable harm. The case settled for $850,000 based on Sandra's detailed analysis connecting device design flaws to patient injury.

Pharmaceutical product liability cases involve adverse drug reactions, manufacturing defects, and inadequate warnings about medication risks. These cases require understanding drug mechanisms, clinical trial data, and regulatory approval processes that determine manufacturer liability for patient harm.

The opioid epidemic generated massive pharmaceutical litigation examining marketing practices, addiction potential disclosure, and prescribing guideline development. Legal nurse consultants with pain management and addiction medicine backgrounds became essential for analyzing complex cases involving multiple pharmaceutical companies and thousands of affected patients.

Implantable device complications create specialized litigation requiring understanding of device insertion procedures, monitoring requirements, and complication management protocols. Pacemakers, defibrillators, insulin pumps, and spinal cord stimulators can malfunction in ways that cause serious patient harm or death.

Former cardiac care nurse Michael Rodriguez analyzed a case involving pacemaker malfunction that caused syncopal episodes and emergency room visits over six months before the device problem was recognized. His analysis showed that typical monitoring protocols should have identified the device failure much earlier, preventing multiple dangerous episodes.

Michael's expertise in cardiac monitoring and pacemaker function helped attorneys understand the technical aspects of device failure while demonstrating how proper monitoring would have prevented patient harm. His analysis contributed to a $1.2 million settlement for the patient's injuries and ongoing cardiac complications.

Toxic Torts and Environmental Health Cases

Environmental exposure litigation requires understanding how chemical, biological, and radiological agents cause human health effects through occupational, residential, or community exposure pathways. These cases often involve multiple plaintiffs with similar exposure histories and health outcomes.

Asbestos litigation continues generating significant case volumes decades after exposure risks became widely known. Mesothelioma, lung cancer, and asbestosis cases require medical experts who understand disease mechanisms, exposure assessment, and latency periods between exposure and disease development.

Chemical exposure analysis focuses on toxicology principles, dose-response relationships, and biological mechanisms connecting environmental exposures to specific health outcomes. You'll need to understand how chemicals enter the body, distribute to target organs, and cause cellular damage that manifests as disease.

Former occupational health nurse Patricia Chen specialized in chemical exposure cases after working in industrial healthcare settings where she observed patterns of work-related illness. Her experience with chemical safety protocols and health surveillance programs provided unique qualifications for toxic tort litigation.

Patricia analyzed a case involving groundwater contamination from an industrial facility that affected a residential community of 200 families. Multiple residents developed similar symptoms— neurological problems, reproductive issues, and immune system dysfunction—after drinking contaminated well water for several years.

Her analysis required understanding the specific chemicals involved (trichloroethylene and perchloroethylene), their toxicological properties, and health effects documented in occupational and environmental health literature. Patricia correlated exposure timelines with symptom development patterns to establish causation connections between contamination and health problems.

The case required Patricia to review extensive environmental monitoring data, health surveillance records, and medical literature establishing biological mechanisms for the observed health effects. Her analysis helped attorneys understand complex toxicology concepts while maintaining focus on human health impacts and community harm. The case resulted in a $45 million settlement covering medical monitoring and compensation for affected residents.

Mass tort litigation involving environmental exposures typically includes hundreds or thousands of plaintiffs with similar exposure histories but varying health outcomes. These cases require systematic analysis approaches that can process large volumes of medical and exposure data efficiently.

Radiation exposure cases from medical procedures, occupational exposures, or environmental releases require understanding radiation physics, biological effects, and dose-response relationships that determine health risks. CT scan overexposure, nuclear facility accidents, and radiotherapy errors generate litigation requiring specialized medical knowledge.

Cancer clusters near industrial facilities often involve complex epidemiological analysis requiring understanding of cancer biology, environmental pathways, and statistical methods for establishing causation connections between exposures and disease patterns.

Workers' Compensation Medical Reviews

Occupational injury analysis requires understanding workplace hazards, injury mechanisms, and work-relatedness determination for various medical conditions. Workers' compensation systems provide benefits for job-related injuries and illnesses, but causation questions often require medical expert analysis.

Repetitive strain injuries, chemical exposures, noise-induced hearing loss, and psychological trauma can all result from workplace conditions. Your role involves analyzing medical evidence to determine if conditions reasonably relate to job duties and work environment exposures.

Causation determination in workers' compensation cases often involves pre-existing conditions aggravated by work activities. The legal standard typically requires work activities to be a "substantial contributing factor" rather than the sole cause of medical problems.

Former emergency nurse Jennifer Williams transitioned to workers' compensation medical review after gaining experience with occupational injuries in the emergency department. Her familiarity with injury patterns and treatment protocols helped insurance companies and attorneys evaluate claim validity and appropriate compensation levels.

Jennifer analyzed a case involving a warehouse worker who developed chronic back pain after lifting injuries over several years. The medical records showed previous back problems from a motor vehicle accident five years earlier, but the worker claimed his job duties significantly worsened his condition.

Her analysis required understanding biomechanics of lifting, degenerative spine disease progression, and medical evidence showing work-related aggravation versus natural disease progression. Jennifer reviewed ergonomic assessments, job descriptions, and medical imaging to determine the extent of work-related contribution to the current disability.

The case required distinguishing between pre-existing degenerative changes and new injuries attributable to work activities. Jennifer's analysis showed that while the worker had previous back problems, the repetitive lifting requirements of his job significantly accelerated disc degeneration and caused additional structural damage beyond normal disease progression.

Psychiatric injury claims in workers' compensation involve stress-related conditions, post-traumatic stress disorder, and depression resulting from workplace incidents or conditions. These cases require understanding psychological causation and treatment requirements for work-related mental health conditions.

Occupational disease cases involve illnesses that develop gradually from workplace exposures to chemicals, dusts, noise, or other hazardous agents. Lung diseases from dust exposure, hearing loss from noise, and cancer from chemical exposures require specialized medical analysis connecting workplace conditions to disease development.

Return-to-work assessments help determine when injured workers can safely resume job duties and what limitations might be necessary to prevent re-injury. These evaluations require understanding both medical restrictions and job requirements to make appropriate recommendations.

Criminal Cases with Medical Components

Medical evidence in criminal cases requires analyzing injury patterns, cause of death determination, and healthcare provider actions in cases involving alleged criminal behavior. Child abuse, elder abuse, domestic violence, and healthcare fraud cases often need medical expert analysis.

Shaken baby syndrome cases involve complex medical evidence about brain injury mechanisms, timing of injuries, and alternative explanations for infant brain damage. These cases require understanding pediatric anatomy, biomechanics of head trauma, and differential diagnosis considerations.

Healthcare fraud investigations involve billing irregularities, unnecessary procedures, and documentation falsification that might constitute criminal behavior. Medicare fraud, prescription drug diversion, and healthcare identity theft cases require medical experts who understand both clinical standards and billing requirements.

Former pediatric nurse Dr. Susan Taylor specialized in child abuse cases after completing additional training in forensic nursing and child protection. Her clinical experience with injured children provided crucial background for analyzing suspected abuse cases in criminal proceedings.

Susan analyzed a case involving a three-month-old infant who arrived at the emergency department with seizures, vomiting, and altered consciousness. CT scans revealed subdural hematoma and retinal hemorrhages that medical staff suspected indicated abusive head trauma.

Her analysis required understanding normal infant development, accident injury patterns versus abusive trauma, and alternative medical explanations for the observed injuries. Susan reviewed medical literature on accidental versus inflicted head trauma in infants while maintaining objectivity about causation determination.

The case required Susan to explain complex medical concepts to prosecutors, defense attorneys, and potentially jury members without medical backgrounds. Her analysis helped legal professionals understand the medical evidence while acknowledging limitations and uncertainties in determining injury mechanisms.

Drug-related criminal cases often involve medical evidence about impairment, addiction, and treatment requirements for substance abuse disorders. DUI cases, prescription fraud, and drug trafficking prosecutions might require medical expert testimony about pharmacology and addiction medicine.

Homicide investigations sometimes require medical analysis of autopsy findings, injury patterns, and cause of death determination. Understanding trauma mechanisms, toxicology results, and time of death estimation can provide crucial evidence in criminal prosecutions.

Professional license violations involving healthcare providers might include criminal charges related to patient harm, prescription drug diversion, or healthcare fraud. These cases require medical experts who understand both clinical standards and regulatory requirements for healthcare professionals.

Elder Care and Nursing Home Litigation

Nursing home negligence cases involve systematic care failures affecting vulnerable elderly residents who cannot advocate for themselves effectively. Pressure ulcers, falls, medication errors, and neglect cases require understanding geriatric care standards and institutional policies.

Staffing inadequacy often underlies multiple care failures in nursing home settings. Understanding nurse-to-patient ratios, skill mix requirements, and care planning standards helps identify systematic problems that contribute to resident harm.

Pressure ulcer litigation requires understanding wound development, staging systems, prevention protocols, and treatment standards for different ulcer severities. Stage III and IV pressure ulcers often indicate serious neglect because proper prevention and early intervention can prevent progression to advanced stages.

Former geriatric nurse Margaret Davis built her practice around nursing home litigation after observing care quality problems during her clinical career. Her experience with dementia care, fall prevention, and medication management provided specialized knowledge for elder care cases.

Margaret analyzed a case involving an 84-year-old nursing home resident who developed multiple stage IV pressure ulcers leading to sepsis and death. The facility claimed the patient's medical conditions and limited mobility made pressure ulcers unavoidable despite appropriate care.

Her analysis revealed systematic care failures including inadequate turning schedules, missing wound assessments, poor nutrition support, and delayed medical interventions. Margaret's review of nursing documentation showed sporadic repositioning, generic care plan entries, and failure to notify physicians about wound deterioration.

The case required Margaret to research pressure ulcer prevention guidelines, analyze facility policies versus actual care provided, and demonstrate how proper interventions could have prevented the devastating wounds. Her analysis showed clear negligence patterns that contributed to preventable suffering and death.

Medication management failures in nursing homes often involve multiple residents receiving inappropriate medications, dangerous drug combinations, or inadequate monitoring for adverse effects. Antipsychotic medications used for behavior control in dementia patients represent a particular area of regulatory concern and litigation.

Fall prevention programs in nursing homes require understanding risk assessment tools, environmental modifications, and intervention strategies that reduce fall risks for elderly residents. Falls with injuries often indicate failures in assessment, care planning, or intervention implementation.

Wandering and elopement cases involve residents with dementia who leave facilities unsupervised and suffer injuries or death. These cases require understanding dementia care standards, facility security requirements, and supervision protocols for cognitively impaired residents.

Family Law Cases Requiring Medical Expertise

Child custody evaluations sometimes require medical expertise about children's health needs, treatment requirements, and parental capacity to provide appropriate medical care. Chronic illnesses, mental health conditions, and special needs children create custody considerations requiring medical analysis.

Medical decision-making authority in custody cases involves understanding treatment options, parental rights, and children's best interests regarding healthcare decisions. Disputes about vaccination, mental health treatment, or experimental therapies might require medical expert input.

Personal injury in family law often involves domestic violence cases requiring medical analysis of injury patterns, healing timelines, and psychological trauma effects. Understanding injury mechanisms helps distinguish between accidental injuries and intentional harm patterns.

Former psychiatric nurse Dr. Linda Foster specialized in family law cases involving mental health issues after developing expertise in child and adolescent psychiatry. Her clinical background provided valuable perspectives on family dynamics and mental health treatment needs.

Linda analyzed a custody case involving a 12-year-old child with attention deficit hyperactivity disorder (ADHD) whose parents disagreed about medication treatment. One parent supported stimulant medication while the other preferred behavioral interventions only.

Her analysis required reviewing the child's medical history, school performance records, and treatment response data to assess the necessity and effectiveness of different intervention approaches. Linda's evaluation considered both the medical literature on ADHD treatment and the specific child's individual needs and responses.

The case required Linda to explain ADHD as a medical condition, review evidence-based treatment options, and provide objective analysis of the child's treatment needs without advocating for either parent's position. Her neutral medical perspective helped the court make informed decisions about the child's healthcare needs.

Reproductive health issues in family law might involve fertility treatment disputes, pregnancy-related medical decisions, or genetic testing considerations affecting custody or support arrangements. Understanding reproductive medicine and genetic counseling helps analyze these complex situations.

Disability determinations for support calculation purposes require medical analysis of functional limitations, treatment requirements, and prognosis for various medical conditions. Social Security disability standards and vocational rehabilitation potential often influence family law financial arrangements.

Substance abuse evaluations in custody cases require understanding addiction medicine, treatment options, and recovery prognosis for parents with substance use disorders. Medical monitoring and treatment compliance become important factors in custody and visitation determinations.

Broadening Your Professional Horizon

Expanding beyond traditional medical malpractice opens opportunities for specialized practice development that offers both intellectual challenge and financial rewards. These diverse practice areas allow you to apply your nursing knowledge in contexts that appreciate your clinical perspective while reducing competition from generalist legal nurse consultants.

86

Each specialty requires dedicated learning and relationship building with attorneys who handle these case types. However, the investment in specialized knowledge often results in premium compensation and more interesting cases that provide professional satisfaction beyond traditional malpractice review.

Practice Expansion Opportunities for Success

- Medical device litigation requires understanding device function, failure mechanisms, and patient symptom patterns for products liability cases

- Toxic tort cases involve environmental exposures requiring toxicology knowledge and health effect analysis for mass litigation

- Workers' compensation medical review focuses on occupational injury causation and work-relatedness determination for insurance claims

- Criminal cases with medical components require objective analysis of injury patterns, causation, and healthcare evidence for prosecution or defense

- Elder care litigation addresses nursing home negligence through geriatric care standards and institutional policy analysis

- Family law medical issues involve child custody, personal injury, and disability evaluations requiring neutral medical expertise

Chapter 8: Emerging High-Value Specializations

The legal implications of healthcare technology advancement create entirely new categories of litigation requiring specialized medical knowledge that traditional legal nurse consultants often lack. You stand at the forefront of emerging practice areas where attorneys desperately need experts who understand both clinical care and technological complexities that shape modern healthcare delivery.

These cutting-edge specializations offer premium compensation because few consultants possess the technical knowledge and clinical experience necessary for effective analysis. Early entry into these emerging fields positions you for substantial practice growth as litigation volumes increase over the next decade.

Telehealth and Remote Care Litigation

Telehealth malpractice represents rapidly expanding litigation as virtual care becomes mainstream healthcare delivery. The pandemic's forced adoption of remote consultation created numerous liability questions about diagnostic accuracy, technology limitations, and appropriate care standards for virtual patient encounters.

Remote diagnosis challenges create unique legal issues when providers cannot perform physical examinations, observe patient appearance directly, or access point-of-care testing that might be available in traditional office settings. Standard care expectations must adapt to technology constraints while maintaining patient safety.

Technology failure liability emerges when communication problems, software glitches, or connectivity issues interfere with patient care delivery. Attorneys need medical experts who understand both clinical requirements and technical limitations that might excuse diagnostic errors or treatment delays.

Former emergency medicine nurse practitioner Dr. Robert Kim built his telehealth litigation practice after providing virtual urgent care during the COVID-19 pandemic. His dual experience in traditional emergency medicine and telehealth delivery provided unique qualifications for analyzing virtual care standard violations.

Robert analyzed a case involving a 45-year-old patient who contacted a telehealth service with chest pain complaints but was advised to take antacids and follow up with primary care. The patient suffered massive myocardial infarction six hours later, requiring emergency cardiac intervention and resulting in permanent heart damage.

His analysis required understanding telehealth evaluation protocols, chest pain assessment standards, and technology limitations affecting diagnostic accuracy. Robert reviewed the virtual consultation recording, provider documentation, and established guidelines for remote cardiac risk assessment.

The case required distinguishing between acceptable telehealth limitations and clear care standard violations. Robert's analysis showed that while telehealth cannot replicate complete physical examination, established protocols require immediate emergency department referral for any chest pain in middle-aged patients regardless of technology constraints.

Prescription management through telehealth platforms creates liability issues when providers prescribe medications without adequate patient evaluation, fail to review drug interactions, or prescribe controlled substances inappropriately. These cases require understanding both telemedicine regulations and prescribing standards.

Remote monitoring device failures involve wearable devices, home monitoring equipment, and smartphone applications that collect patient data for clinical decision-making. When these technologies malfunction or provide inaccurate data, patient harm might result from inappropriate treatment decisions.

The case analyzed by former cardiac care nurse Jennifer Martinez involved a patient with heart failure whose remote monitoring device failed to transmit weight gain data indicating fluid retention. The patient was hospitalized with pulmonary edema that might have been prevented with proper monitoring and medication adjustment.

Jennifer's analysis required understanding heart failure management protocols, remote monitoring technology capabilities, and appropriate response systems for device failure alerts. Her expertise in both cardiac care and monitoring technology helped attorneys understand the complex interaction between clinical care and technology systems.

AI Diagnostic Failure Cases

Artificial intelligence diagnostic errors create new liability categories when algorithmic systems fail to identify diseases, provide incorrect diagnoses, or recommend inappropriate treatments. These cases require understanding both clinical diagnostic processes and AI system limitations that contribute to patient harm.

Machine learning diagnostic systems analyze medical images, laboratory data, and clinical symptoms to generate diagnostic recommendations or risk assessments. When these systems fail, attorneys need experts who understand both the medical conditions involved and the technology's decision-making processes.

Algorithm bias and discrimination issues emerge when AI systems perform differently for various patient populations, potentially missing diseases in women, minorities, or elderly patients. These cases require understanding both clinical epidemiology and machine learning bias sources.

Former radiology nurse turned informatics specialist Dr. Patricia Williams specialized in AI diagnostic failure cases after working with computerized diagnostic systems in her clinical career. Her understanding of both clinical decision-making and technology implementation provided unique qualifications for AI litigation.

Patricia analyzed a case involving an AI mammography screening system that failed to identify early-stage breast cancer in a 52-year-old woman. The cancer progressed to advanced stages before clinical detection, requiring extensive treatment that might have been avoided with earlier diagnosis.

Her analysis required understanding mammography interpretation standards, AI image analysis capabilities, and factors that might cause algorithm failures. Patricia reviewed the AI system's training data, performance statistics, and quality assurance procedures to identify potential causes of the diagnostic failure.

The case required distinguishing between acceptable AI system limitations and clear failures to meet diagnostic standards. Patricia's analysis showed that while AI systems have inherent limitations, this particular failure occurred despite clear radiographic evidence that should have triggered cancer detection alerts.

Clinical decision support failures involve computerized systems that provide treatment recommendations, drug interaction warnings, or clinical guideline reminders. When these systems malfunction or provide inappropriate advice, patient harm might result from following incorrect algorithmic recommendations.

Data input errors affecting AI diagnostic accuracy create liability questions about system design, user interface adequacy, and quality control procedures that should prevent incorrect data from reaching algorithmic decision-making systems.

Medical device AI integration failures involve diagnostic equipment that incorporates artificial intelligence for image interpretation, rhythm analysis, or parameter calculation. When these integrated systems fail, determining liability between device manufacturers and software developers requires specialized technical knowledge.

Healthcare Cybersecurity Breaches

Ransomware attack consequences on healthcare systems create patient care disruptions that might result in treatment delays, medication errors, or diagnostic failures. When cybersecurity incidents affect clinical operations, attorneys need medical experts who understand both care requirements and technology dependencies.

Hospital information systems control medication administration, laboratory reporting, imaging systems, and electronic health records that are essential for safe patient care. Cyber attacks that disrupt these systems can cause widespread care quality problems with serious patient safety implications.

Electronic health record disruptions during cybersecurity incidents might cause providers to lose access to patient medical histories, medication lists, and critical clinical information needed for safe care decisions. These disruptions can cause errors that might not occur with normal system access.

Former chief nursing informatics officer Dr. Lisa Park specialized in cybersecurity litigation after managing hospital responses to multiple cyber attacks. Her experience with clinical system operations and emergency response procedures provided unique qualifications for analyzing cyber incident patient care effects.

Lisa analyzed a case involving a major hospital ransomware attack that disrupted electronic systems for five days, forcing providers to use paper documentation and manual processes. Several patients experienced medication errors, delayed treatments, and missed diagnoses during the system disruption period.

Her analysis required understanding normal clinical workflows, manual backup procedures, and patient safety protocols during technology failures. Lisa reviewed incident reports, temporary documentation systems, and patient care outcomes to identify preventable harm resulting from inadequate cyber incident response.

The case required distinguishing between unavoidable technology disruption effects and preventable care failures resulting from inadequate emergency response planning. Lisa's analysis showed that while cyber attacks create inherent challenges, proper backup procedures and staff training could have prevented most of the observed patient safety incidents.

Medical device cybersecurity vulnerabilities create risks when networked clinical equipment becomes compromised through cyber attacks. Infusion pumps, patient monitors, and diagnostic equipment connected to hospital networks might be vulnerable to malicious interference that affects patient care.

Patient data breach consequences might not directly cause physical harm but can result in identity theft, discrimination, or psychological trauma requiring compensation. Understanding the scope and impact of healthcare data breaches helps attorneys evaluate appropriate damage calculations.

Protected health information theft for fraud purposes can cause patients significant financial and emotional harm requiring legal remediation. Medical identity theft might result in incorrect medical information entering patient records, potentially affecting future care decisions and insurance coverage.

Mental Health and Psychiatric Nursing Cases

Psychiatric medication errors create serious liability issues because psychotropic medications often have narrow therapeutic windows, dangerous drug interactions, and potentially life-threatening side effects that require careful monitoring and dose adjustment.

Suicide prevention failures in healthcare settings require understanding risk assessment protocols, safety procedures, and monitoring standards that should prevent self-harm in vulnerable patients. These cases involve analyzing both clinical judgment and institutional policies.

Involuntary commitment procedures create legal issues when patients are held against their will without proper legal authority or when dangerous patients are inappropriately discharged. Understanding mental health laws and clinical assessment standards helps analyze these complex cases.

Former psychiatric nurse Dr. Michael Rodriguez specialized in mental health litigation after 20 years of experience in inpatient psychiatric settings. His clinical background in crisis intervention and suicide prevention provided essential qualifications for psychiatric nursing standard analysis.

Michael analyzed a case involving a 28-year-old patient who committed suicide 12 hours after discharge from a hospital emergency department following a psychiatric evaluation. The family alleged that inadequate risk assessment and premature discharge caused the preventable death.

His analysis required understanding suicide risk assessment tools, emergency psychiatric evaluation standards, and discharge planning requirements for suicidal patients. Michael reviewed the psychiatric consultation documentation, nursing assessments, and established protocols for suicide risk management.

The case required analyzing both clinical judgment quality and adherence to established psychiatric care standards. Michael's analysis showed that while suicide prediction remains imperfect, the emergency department evaluation failed to adequately assess known risk factors and ignored family concerns about the patient's safety.

Psychiatric emergency care in general hospital settings often involves inadequate training, insufficient resources, and inappropriate treatment that falls below psychiatric nursing standards. Medical-surgical nurses caring for psychiatric patients might lack specialized knowledge needed for safe care.

Psychotropic medication monitoring requires understanding complex drug interactions, side effect profiles, and laboratory monitoring requirements that differ significantly from general medical medications. Failure to provide appropriate monitoring can result in serious patient harm or death.

Electroconvulsive therapy complications require specialized knowledge about anesthesia procedures, seizure monitoring, and recovery protocols that differ from other medical procedures. ECT-related injuries might result from inadequate anesthesia, positioning errors, or recovery monitoring failures.

Pharmaceutical and Clinical Trial Litigation

Drug approval fraud cases involve pharmaceutical companies that allegedly concealed safety data, manipulated clinical trial results, or failed to disclose known adverse effects during FDA approval processes. These cases require understanding both clinical research methods and regulatory approval requirements.

Clinical trial participant injury litigation requires understanding informed consent requirements, research protocols, and investigator responsibilities for participant safety. When research subjects suffer harm from experimental treatments, determining liability requires specialized knowledge about research ethics and safety standards.

Off-label prescribing liability emerges when physicians prescribe approved medications for unapproved uses that result in patient harm. Understanding drug approval processes, clinical evidence standards, and prescribing practices helps analyze these complex cases.

Former clinical research nurse Dr. Sandra Chen specialized in pharmaceutical litigation after coordinating clinical trials for major pharmaceutical companies. Her experience with research protocols and drug development provided unique qualifications for analyzing research-related liability issues.

Sandra analyzed a case involving a clinical trial participant who developed liver failure while taking an experimental arthritis medication. The patient alleged that the research team failed to provide adequate safety monitoring and ignored early warning signs of hepatic toxicity.

Her analysis required understanding clinical trial protocols, safety monitoring requirements, and adverse event reporting procedures for experimental drugs. Sandra reviewed the research protocol, informed consent documents, and safety monitoring reports to identify potential violations of research standards.

The case required analyzing both research protocol compliance and clinical judgment about participant safety. Sandra's analysis showed that while experimental drug development involves inherent risks, the research team failed to follow established safety monitoring procedures and ignored laboratory abnormalities that should have triggered immediate intervention.

Post-market surveillance failures involve pharmaceutical companies that fail to adequately monitor drug safety after FDA approval or delay reporting adverse effects to regulatory authorities. These cases require understanding pharmacovigilance requirements and post-market safety obligations.

Generic drug quality issues create liability when manufacturing problems result in contaminated medications, incorrect formulations, or packaging errors that cause patient harm. Understanding pharmaceutical manufacturing standards and quality control procedures helps analyze these cases.

Drug interaction lawsuits often involve multiple pharmaceutical companies when combination therapies result in dangerous interactions that cause patient harm. Determining relative liability requires understanding drug metabolism, interaction mechanisms, and labeling requirements.

COVID-Related Healthcare Litigation

Pandemic care standards created unique legal issues when healthcare systems operated under crisis conditions with limited resources, modified protocols, and emergency regulatory changes. Determining appropriate care standards during healthcare emergencies requires understanding both normal expectations and crisis modifications.

Ventilator allocation decisions during equipment shortages raised ethical and legal questions about resource distribution and patient selection criteria. These cases require understanding both clinical factors affecting treatment decisions and institutional policies for resource allocation.

Personal protective equipment failures caused healthcare worker infections and deaths when employers failed to provide adequate protection or required workers to reuse single-use equipment. These cases involve both occupational safety standards and healthcare worker protection requirements.

Former intensive care nurse Dr. Jennifer Washington specialized in COVID-related litigation after working in ICU settings throughout the pandemic. Her experience with crisis care protocols and resource limitations provided unique qualifications for analyzing pandemic-related liability issues.

Jennifer analyzed a case involving a healthcare worker who developed severe COVID-19 after being required to reuse N95 masks for an entire week due to supply shortages. The worker required prolonged ICU care and suffered permanent lung damage affecting future work capacity.

Her analysis required understanding infection control standards, personal protective equipment effectiveness, and occupational safety requirements during healthcare emergencies. Jennifer reviewed hospital policies, supply chain documentation, and regulatory guidance about PPE conservation strategies.

The case required analyzing both emergency modifications to normal standards and employer obligations to protect healthcare workers. Jennifer's analysis showed that while pandemic conditions created unprecedented challenges, the hospital's PPE conservation policies violated established infection control principles and worker safety requirements.

Vaccine administration errors during mass vaccination campaigns created liability issues when healthcare workers administered incorrect doses, wrong vaccines, or failed to follow proper screening procedures. Understanding vaccination protocols and emergency use authorization requirements helps analyze these cases.

Long COVID disability claims require understanding the evolving medical knowledge about persistent symptoms, functional limitations, and treatment options for post-acute COVID syndrome. These cases involve complex medical causation analysis and disability assessment.

Nursing home COVID outbreaks generated extensive litigation when facilities failed to implement adequate infection control measures, leading to widespread resident infections and deaths. Understanding long-term care standards and infection prevention requirements helps analyze institutional liability.

The Future of Legal Medicine

Emerging healthcare technologies and changing practice patterns create new opportunities for legal nurse consultants who position themselves at the intersection of clinical knowledge and technological understanding. These specialized practice areas offer both intellectual challenges and financial rewards that exceed traditional malpractice consulting.

The key to success in emerging specializations lies in combining your clinical foundation with focused learning about new technologies and their legal implications. Early entry into these developing fields provides competitive advantages that can establish lasting professional recognition and premium compensation.

Specialized Practice Development for Tomorrow's Market

- Telehealth litigation requires understanding virtual care standards and technology limitations affecting diagnostic accuracy and treatment delivery

- AI diagnostic failure cases need expertise in both clinical decision-making and algorithmic system limitations that contribute to patient harm

- Healthcare cybersecurity breach analysis demands knowledge of clinical workflows and technology dependencies that affect patient safety

- Mental health litigation requires specialized psychiatric nursing knowledge and understanding of complex medication monitoring requirements

- Pharmaceutical and clinical trial cases involve research protocol compliance and drug development safety standards beyond general medical knowledge

- COVID-related litigation addresses pandemic care modifications and resource allocation decisions during healthcare emergencies

Chapter 9: From Consultant to Expert Witness

The transition from case consultant to expert witness represents both the pinnacle of legal nurse consulting success and its most demanding challenge. Expert witness work commands premium compensation ($250-400 per hour) but requires exceptional qualifications, advanced communication skills, and the ability to defend your opinions under aggressive cross-examination from opposing attorneys.

This professional evolution demands more than clinical expertise—you must develop courtroom presence, master complex legal procedures, and maintain credibility under intense scrutiny that can make or break million-dollar cases. The rewards justify the challenges for consultants who develop the specialized skills that separate expert witnesses from general consultants.

When Attorneys Need Expert Testimony vs Consultation

Consultation services provide behind-the-scenes analysis that helps attorneys understand medical issues, evaluate case merit, and develop litigation strategies without appearing in court or providing formal opinions about care standards. Consultants work confidentially as part of the legal team's internal case development process.

Attorney work product protection shields consultation activities from discovery by opposing counsel, allowing frank discussions about case weaknesses, alternative theories, and strategic considerations. This confidential relationship enables thorough case analysis without concern about opposing attorney access to internal assessments.

Expert witness testimony provides formal opinions about care standards, causation, and damages that become part of the official court record and are subject to discovery by opposing counsel. Expert witnesses must disclose their opinions, supporting materials, and compensation arrangements as part of the litigation process.

The decision between consultation and expert testimony often depends on case strategy, evidence strength, and available expert qualifications. Strong cases with clear liability might proceed directly to expert testimony, while complex cases with unclear outcomes benefit from confidential consultation before committing to expert witness designation.

Case strength assessment helps attorneys determine the appropriate level of expert involvement based on evidence quality and likelihood of successful outcome. Weak cases might benefit from consultation to identify problems before investing in expensive expert witness preparation and testimony.

Former surgical nurse Dr. Patricia Thompson learned this lesson when an attorney asked her to serve as expert witness in a surgical malpractice case that she had initially evaluated as consultant. Her confidential analysis revealed significant case weaknesses that made expert testimony inadvisable despite clear medical issues.

Patricia's consultation showed that while surgical technique problems existed, the patient's pre-existing conditions and post-operative compliance issues created causation challenges that opposing experts could exploit effectively. She recommended additional medical evaluation before proceeding with expert witness designation.

The attorney ultimately declined the case based on Patricia's consultation, avoiding expensive litigation with poor prospects for success. This example illustrates how consultation services protect attorneys from pursuing cases that appear strong initially but have hidden weaknesses that expert analysis reveals.

Discovery obligations for expert witnesses include providing detailed reports outlining all opinions, supporting materials, and reasoning processes. These reports become roadmaps for opposing counsel cross-examination and must withstand careful scrutiny for consistency and accuracy.

Consultation confidentiality allows attorneys to explore multiple theories, consider alternative approaches, and develop case strategy without creating discoverable materials that opposing counsel can access. This protection enables thorough case development without strategic disclosure to opponents.

Expert witness reports typically include detailed qualifications statements, case summaries, records reviewed, literature researched, opinions formed, and supporting reasoning. These comprehensive documents often exceed 20-30 pages for complex cases and require careful preparation to avoid creating cross-examination vulnerabilities.

Qualification Requirements and Credibility Building

Educational foundation for expert witness qualification typically requires minimum bachelor's degree in nursing, though many courts prefer advanced degrees that demonstrate specialized knowledge and academic achievement. Master's and doctoral degrees in relevant specialties strengthen qualification arguments and credibility assessment.

Clinical experience requirements vary by case type but generally require minimum 5-10 years of hands-on practice in areas relevant to the litigation. Recent experience proves more valuable than distant historical practice because care standards and technology change rapidly in healthcare settings.

Certification credentials from recognized professional organizations enhance expert witness qualifications and demonstrate ongoing competence in specialized practice areas. CCRN certification for critical care cases, CEN certification for emergency medicine, and other specialty certifications support expert qualification arguments.

The Legal Nurse Consultant Certified (LNCC) credential from the American Association of Legal Nurse Consultants represents the gold standard for legal nurse consulting expertise, though it requires 2,000 hours of LNC experience plus rigorous examination passage.

Teaching and publication experience strengthens expert witness credibility by demonstrating knowledge sharing and peer recognition within professional communities. University faculty appointments, conference presentations, and peer-reviewed publications provide evidence of expertise beyond clinical practice.

Dr. Michael Rodriguez built his expert witness credentials systematically after transitioning from emergency nursing to legal consulting. He completed a master's degree in nursing administration, maintained CEN certification, published articles about emergency care standards, and taught emergency nursing courses at a local university.

His qualification portfolio included 15 years of emergency department experience, five years of legal nurse consulting, advanced certification in emergency nursing, three published articles about emergency care protocols, and adjunct faculty experience teaching emergency assessment skills.

The systematic credential building allowed Michael to qualify as expert witness in emergency medicine cases where his combination of clinical experience, legal knowledge, and academic credentials provided compelling qualification arguments that courts accepted without challenge.

Continuing education requirements for expert witnesses include staying current with clinical practice standards, legal developments, and professional literature that affects testimony areas. Formal continuing education credits demonstrate ongoing competence and knowledge updates.

Previous testimony experience becomes self-reinforcing because courts and attorneys prefer expert witnesses with proven courtroom performance and cross-examination survival skills. Building initial testimony experience requires accepting cases at reduced compensation to develop courtroom skills and track record.

Professional liability insurance for expert witness activities provides financial protection against malpractice claims related to testimony quality, opinion accuracy, and professional conduct during litigation. Standard nursing malpractice insurance typically excludes expert witness activities, requiring specialized coverage.

Deposition Preparation and Performance

Deposition purpose in expert witness proceedings serves multiple functions: preserving testimony for trial use, allowing opposing counsel to evaluate witness qualifications and opinions, and providing discovery of expert reasoning and supporting materials.

Opposing attorneys use depositions to assess witness credibility, identify opinion weaknesses, and develop cross-examination strategies for trial proceedings. Effective deposition performance can strengthen your position while poor performance might eliminate you from the case entirely.

Preparation strategies require thorough review of all case materials, supporting literature, and previous testimony transcripts to ensure consistency and accuracy throughout the deposition process. Any inconsistencies between deposition testimony and trial testimony can devastate witness credibility.

Attorney preparation sessions help identify potential problem areas, practice difficult questions, and develop clear explanations for complex medical concepts that non-medical audiences can understand. These practice sessions often reveal opinion weaknesses that require additional research or clarification.

Question anticipation involves considering all possible challenges to your opinions, alternative explanations for case facts, and potential attacks on your qualifications or methodology. Experienced opposing counsel will probe every aspect of your analysis looking for weaknesses or contradictions.

Former ICU nurse Dr. Jennifer Martinez learned effective deposition techniques through experience with aggressive opposing counsel who challenged every aspect of her critical care expertise. Her first deposition involved medication error case where opposing counsel questioned her pharmacology knowledge, unit policies familiarity, and quality improvement experience.

The challenging experience taught Jennifer to prepare more thoroughly, research supporting literature extensively, and practice clear explanations for complex critical care concepts. Her improved preparation led to confident deposition performance that strengthened her position in subsequent trial proceedings.

Documentation review before depositions requires re-reading all case records, expert reports, and supporting materials to ensure accurate recall of specific details. Deposition questioning often focuses on minute details that can affect overall opinion credibility if recalled incorrectly.

Professional demeanor during depositions requires maintaining composure, speaking clearly, and avoiding defensive responses to aggressive questioning. Calm, confident responses project competence while emotional reactions suggest uncertainty or weakness in opinion foundation.

Listen to questions carefully and answer only what is asked without volunteering additional information that might create new areas for opposing counsel exploration. "I don't know" or "I don't recall" are acceptable responses when information is genuinely unavailable or forgotten.

Courtroom Testimony Best Practices

Direct examination by retaining counsel provides opportunity to present your qualifications, explain your opinions, and educate the jury about relevant medical concepts in supportive environment with friendly questioning designed to highlight your expertise.

Qualification testimony establishes your credibility through education, experience, and professional achievements that demonstrate expertise in case-relevant areas. This foundation determines whether the court accepts you as expert witness qualified to provide opinion testimony.

Opinion presentation requires clear, logical explanations that guide non-medical audiences through complex medical reasoning without overwhelming them with technical details. Use analogies, visual aids, and simple language to make concepts accessible to jury understanding.

Visual presentations including medical illustrations, timeline charts, and demonstration materials help juries understand complex medical concepts and retain key information throughout trial proceedings. Effective visual aids can determine jury comprehension and case outcomes.

Education approach for jury instruction focuses on teaching medical concepts necessary for understanding your opinions rather than advocating for specific legal conclusions. Neutral educational testimony appears more credible than obvious advocacy that might suggest bias.

Dr. Sandra Chen developed effective courtroom teaching techniques during her expert witness career in medication error cases. Her approach involved explaining normal medication administration processes before describing specific errors and their consequences in case-specific situations.

Sandra's testimony began with basic pharmacology education—how medications work, why proper dosing matters, and what safety checks prevent errors. This foundation helped juries understand the significance of care standard violations and their relationship to patient harm.

Her visual aids included medication calculation examples, drug interaction charts, and patient monitoring timelines that illustrated proper procedures versus actual care provided. These educational materials helped juries understand complex medical concepts while maintaining focus on case-specific issues.

Confidence projection through posture, voice quality, and eye contact affects jury perception of witness credibility and opinion reliability. Nervous or uncertain presentations suggest opinion weakness while confident delivery implies expertise and conviction.

Jury connection involves maintaining appropriate eye contact, speaking directly to jurors, and using language that demonstrates respect for their intelligence while ensuring understanding of complex medical concepts.

Medical terminology explanations should be clear and complete without appearing condescending to jury intelligence. Define terms naturally within testimony flow rather than stopping to provide lengthy technical definitions that interrupt reasoning presentation.

Cross-Examination Survival Strategies

Aggressive questioning by opposing counsel aims to discredit your qualifications, challenge opinion accuracy, expose methodology flaws, and create doubt about conclusion reliability. These attacks can be personal, technical, and relentless in pursuing any perceived weakness.

Preparation for cross-examination requires anticipating every possible challenge to your opinions and developing clear, concise responses that maintain opinion credibility while acknowledging appropriate limitations or uncertainties.

Common attack strategies include qualification challenges (questioning education, experience, or certification adequacy), methodology criticism (challenging research methods or analysis approaches), and opinion inconsistency claims (comparing testimony to previous cases or published statements).

Literature attacks involve opposing counsel presenting medical studies or guidelines that appear to contradict your opinions, requiring detailed knowledge of medical literature and ability to explain apparent contradictions or study limitations.

Response strategies for aggressive questioning include staying calm, listening carefully to questions, and providing direct answers without defensive elaboration that might create additional attack opportunities.

Former emergency nurse Dr. Robert Kim survived particularly aggressive cross-examination in a delayed myocardial infarction case where opposing counsel spent four hours challenging his emergency medicine experience, diagnostic reasoning, and opinion consistency with published guidelines.

The opposing attorney questioned Robert's certification maintenance, emergency department policies knowledge, and familiarity with specific cardiac risk assessment tools. Each challenge required detailed responses that demonstrated expertise while avoiding defensive reactions that might suggest uncertainty.

Robert's survival strategy involved thorough preparation, extensive literature review, and practice sessions with retaining counsel that identified potential weaknesses and developed appropriate responses. His calm, knowledgeable responses maintained opinion credibility despite aggressive challenging.

Impeachment attempts occur when opposing counsel presents evidence of prior inconsistent statements, testimony contradictions, or qualification misrepresentations that could destroy witness credibility entirely.

Document traps involve opposing counsel presenting medical records, literature excerpts, or previous testimony quotes out of context to create apparent contradictions with current testimony. Careful document review and context consideration help avoid these traps.

Professional integrity requires honest acknowledgment of opinion limitations, knowledge gaps, and uncertainty areas while maintaining confidence in core opinions. Attempts to appear omniscient usually backfire when opposing counsel exposes knowledge limitations.

Premium Pricing for Expert Witness Services

Hourly compensation for expert witness services ranges from $250-400 per hour for testimony and preparation time, with experienced experts in specialized areas commanding higher rates based on qualifications and track record.

Geographic markets affect compensation levels with major metropolitan areas typically offering higher rates than rural markets. Complex federal cases often pay premium rates compared to state court litigation with smaller damage amounts.

Preparation time billing includes record review, literature research, report writing, attorney consultations, and deposition preparation activities. Experienced experts typically require 40-80 hours of preparation for complex cases requiring detailed analysis and comprehensive reporting.

Testimony time billing covers deposition and trial testimony plus travel time for out-of-town proceedings. Some experts charge portal-to-portal rates while others bill only for actual testimony time depending on client arrangements and market practices.

Retainer requirements help ensure payment for expert witness services that can extend over months or years before case resolution. Typical retainers range from $5,000-15,000 for complex cases requiring extensive preparation and multiple appearances.

Cancellation policies protect expert witness income when cases settle unexpectedly or testimony is cancelled on short notice. Many experts charge cancellation fees for last-minute changes that prevent accepting other cases during reserved time periods.

Dr. Lisa Park developed successful expert witness pricing strategies after learning from early career mistakes that undervalued her expertise and created payment problems with attorney clients.

Her current pricing structure includes $350 per hour for all expert witness activities, minimum retainers of $10,000 for complex cases, and 48-hour cancellation policies that protect against income loss from sudden case changes.

Lisa's premium pricing reflects her specialized credentials in pediatric critical care, extensive courtroom experience with over 50 testimony appearances, and proven track record of helping attorneys achieve successful case outcomes.

Value-based pricing considerations include case complexity, damage amounts at stake, and attorney budget constraints that might affect compensation negotiations. High-value cases typically justify premium expert witness rates while smaller cases might require fee adjustments.

Payment terms for expert witness services typically require monthly invoicing with net 30-day payment terms, though some experts demand faster payment schedules due to cash flow requirements and collection challenges with attorney clients.

Professional collection procedures for unpaid expert witness fees might include attorney referral, collection agency services, or small claims court proceedings depending on amount involved and client relationship considerations.

Reaching Professional Excellence

Expert witness work represents the culmination of legal nurse consulting career development, offering both maximum compensation and greatest professional challenges. Success requires systematic credential building, advanced communication skills, and courtroom presence that develops through experience and dedicated preparation.

The transition from consultant to expert witness requires significant investment in education, training, and relationship building with attorney clients who value exceptional expertise and courtroom effectiveness. However, the financial and professional rewards justify the effort for consultants who achieve expert witness success.

Expert Witness Development Pathway to Success

- Expert testimony differs from consultation through formal opinion requirements and discovery obligations that affect case strategy and attorney relationships

- Qualification building requires systematic credential development including education, certification, experience, and publication activities that establish expertise

- Deposition performance demands thorough preparation and professional demeanor that can strengthen or eliminate expert witness effectiveness

- Courtroom testimony requires educational approach and confidence projection that helps juries understand complex medical concepts

- Cross-examination survival needs aggressive questioning preparation and response strategies that maintain opinion credibility under attack

- Premium pricing reflects specialized expertise and courtroom experience that justifies $250-400 hourly compensation for qualified expert witnesses

Chapter 10: Business Structure and Legal Requirements

The business foundation you establish for your legal nurse consulting practice determines everything from tax obligations to personal liability protection—yet most nurses approach this decision with the same casual planning they'd use for choosing lunch. Your business structure affects liability exposure, tax strategy, professional credibility, and growth potential in ways that compound over years of practice development.

Getting the structure right from the beginning saves money, protects assets, and positions your practice for sustainable growth. Getting it wrong creates expensive problems that can undermine even the most successful consulting practices through unnecessary tax burdens, liability exposure, and credibility challenges with attorney clients.

LLC vs Corporation vs Sole Proprietorship Analysis

Sole proprietorship represents the simplest business structure requiring no formal registration or separate entity creation. You operate as an individual providing services under your own name or a trade name, with business income and expenses reported on your personal tax return using Schedule C.

The simplicity appeals to many new consultants who want to start quickly without legal complexity or registration costs. You can begin accepting clients immediately, deduct business expenses directly, and maintain complete control over all business decisions without corporate formalities.

However, sole proprietorship provides no liability protection between your business activities and personal assets. If a client sues your practice, your home, savings, and other personal property become vulnerable to legal judgments. This exposure creates unacceptable risk for consultants handling sensitive medical information and providing expert opinions in high-stakes litigation.

Limited Liability Company (LLC) structure provides liability protection while maintaining operational flexibility and tax advantages that make it the preferred choice for most legal nurse consulting practices. LLC formation creates a separate legal entity that shields personal assets from business liabilities while avoiding corporate tax complications.

LLC members enjoy "pass-through" taxation where business profits and losses flow directly to personal tax returns without separate corporate tax filings. This structure eliminates double taxation problems while providing expense deduction benefits and retirement plan options that sole proprietors cannot access.

The operational flexibility allows multiple ownership structures, profit distribution arrangements, and management approaches that adapt to changing business needs. You can add partners, change ownership percentages, or modify operating agreements without complex corporate procedures.

Former ICU nurse Dr. Patricia Martinez chose LLC structure when establishing her critical care consulting practice after learning from colleagues' liability experiences. Her decision proved wise when a client sued over expert witness testimony that allegedly caused case dismissal, though the lawsuit ultimately failed.

Patricia's LLC structure protected her personal assets during the litigation while allowing business continuation without interruption. The legal separation between her business entity and personal finances meant the lawsuit couldn't attach to her home, retirement accounts, or other personal property regardless of case outcomes.

Her attorney explained that sole proprietorship would have exposed all personal assets to the claim, potentially forcing bankruptcy despite the frivolous nature of the lawsuit. The LLC protection allowed Patricia to defend the case confidently while maintaining financial security for her family.

Professional Limited Liability Company (PLLC) represents a specialized LLC variant designed for licensed professionals providing services within their professional scope. Some states require PLLC formation for licensed healthcare professionals offering consulting services, while others allow standard LLC formation.

PLLC structure maintains liability protection for business debts and most professional claims while preserving professional licensing requirements and ethical obligations. However, PLLC formation typically cannot protect against professional malpractice claims arising from your nursing expertise and services.

Corporate structure options include C-corporations and S-corporations that provide maximum liability protection and formal business recognition but require complex administrative procedures and potential tax disadvantages for small consulting practices.

C-corporation formation creates separate tax entities subject to corporate income tax plus personal taxes on distributed profits—the "double taxation" problem that reduces overall financial efficiency. S-corporation election avoids double taxation through pass-through structure but restricts ownership and profit distribution flexibility.

The administrative burden includes corporate formalities like regular board meetings, written resolutions, and detailed record-keeping requirements that consume time and resources without corresponding benefits for most legal nurse consulting practices.

State-specific requirements vary significantly for business formation, ongoing compliance, and professional licensing obligations that affect structure selection. Some states impose annual fees, publication requirements, or professional oversight that influence optimal structure choice.

Research your state's specific requirements before making structure decisions, as changing business entities later involves expense and complexity that proper initial planning can avoid.

Professional Liability Insurance Requirements

Professional liability coverage provides financial protection against claims that your consulting services caused client harm through errors, omissions, or professional negligence. Standard homeowner's or business liability policies exclude professional services, requiring specialized coverage for legal nurse consulting activities.

Coverage amounts typically range from $1-2 million per occurrence with annual aggregate limits of $2-4 million depending on practice scope and client requirements. Many attorney clients require minimum coverage verification before engaging consulting services, making adequate insurance necessary for business development.

Legal nurse consulting policies differ from standard nursing malpractice insurance because they cover consulting advice, expert witness testimony, and business activities beyond direct patient care. Standard nursing policies often exclude business consulting and expert witness activities, requiring separate specialized coverage.

The coverage should include legal defense costs for baseless claims, settlement payments for valid claims, and business protection against professional liability lawsuits that could destroy practice finances even if ultimately unsuccessful.

Expert witness coverage represents specialized protection for testimony-related claims that standard consulting policies might exclude. Expert witness activities create higher liability exposure because testimony directly affects case outcomes and damage awards, making specialized coverage essential for witnesses.

Former surgical nurse Dr. Michael Rodriguez learned about expert witness coverage needs when opposing counsel threatened malpractice claims related to his testimony in a surgical case. His standard nursing policy excluded expert witness activities, requiring separate coverage purchase to protect against testimony-related liability.

Michael's expert witness insurer provided legal defense against the frivolous claim while his practice continued without financial disruption. The case demonstrated that expert witnesses face litigation risks beyond traditional nursing practice, requiring specialized insurance protection.

Business liability insurance covers general business operations including premises liability, business personal property, and activities unrelated to professional services. This coverage protects against slip-and-fall claims in your office, equipment theft, and other general business risks.

Cyber liability coverage protects against data breaches, ransomware attacks, and technology failures that could compromise protected health information or business operations. HIPAA compliance requirements make cyber coverage increasingly important for consultants handling medical records.

Errors and omissions coverage specifically addresses professional mistakes that cause client financial harm even without traditional malpractice elements. This coverage protects against claims that your analysis errors caused attorneys to pursue weak cases or miss strong claims.

The coverage should include business interruption protection that replaces lost income during claim investigation and defense periods.

Professional liability lawsuits can prevent client work continuation even when claims lack merit, requiring income replacement during defense periods.

Contract Templates and Negotiation Strategies

Service agreements establish legal relationships between legal nurse consultants and attorney clients while defining scope of work, compensation terms, deliverable requirements, and responsibility limitations. Well-drafted contracts prevent misunderstandings while protecting both parties' interests.

Standard contract elements include service descriptions, payment terms, deadline requirements, confidentiality obligations, liability limitations, and dispute resolution procedures. Each element requires careful consideration to balance client needs with consultant protection and business requirements.

Scope of work definitions prevent "scope creep" where clients expect additional services beyond original agreements without additional compensation. Detailed work descriptions, deliverable specifications, and change order procedures maintain project boundaries and fair compensation.

Independent contractor provisions clarify the consulting relationship while avoiding employment classification problems that could create tax and benefit obligations for attorney clients. Proper contractor language protects both parties from unintended employment relationships.

Former emergency nurse Jennifer Williams developed effective contract templates after early career problems with unclear agreements that led to payment disputes and scope expansion without additional compensation. Her experience taught valuable lessons about contract protection importance.

Jennifer's first major case involved oral agreement for medical record review that expanded to include expert witness preparation, deposition attendance, and trial testimony without compensation discussions. The attorney assumed expanded services were included while Jennifer expected additional payment for extra work.

The dispute damaged their professional relationship and delayed payment for months while they negotiated fair compensation for completed work. Jennifer's experience led to detailed written contracts that specify all services, compensation methods, and change procedures before work begins.

Payment protection clauses include late payment penalties, collection cost recovery, and work stoppage rights that protect consultants from payment delays or non-payment problems. Attorney clients often face cash flow challenges that can affect consultant payment timeliness.

Limitation of liability provisions restrict consultant responsibility for attorney decisions, case outcomes, and consequential damages beyond direct service fees. These limitations protect against claims that consulting errors caused large financial losses through case dismissal or unfavorable outcomes.

Confidentiality and non-disclosure agreements protect attorney work product and case strategies while ensuring appropriate handling of protected health information. These provisions must balance legal confidentiality requirements with HIPAA compliance obligations.

Pricing Strategies: Hourly vs Project vs Retainer

Hourly billing provides the most common and flexible compensation method for legal nurse consulting services, allowing fair payment for varying work complexity and time requirements. Hourly rates typically range from $125-300 depending on experience, specialization, and geographic market conditions.

The hourly approach works well for unpredictable projects like medical record review where document volume and complexity vary significantly between cases. Clients pay only for actual time invested while consultants receive compensation proportional to effort required.

Time tracking accuracy becomes essential for hourly billing credibility and client relationship maintenance. Detailed time records showing specific activities and time increments demonstrate value while protecting against billing disputes or questions about work efficiency.

Professional time tracking software provides detailed record-keeping capabilities with client reporting features that support billing accuracy and dispute resolution. Manual time tracking often proves inadequate for complex cases involving multiple activities and clients.

Project-based pricing offers fixed fees for defined deliverables like medical chronologies, case summaries, or expert reports regardless of time required for completion. This approach provides client cost certainty while allowing consultant efficiency rewards for streamlined work processes.

Project pricing works best for standardized services with predictable scope and complexity. Medical record organization, basic case screening, and routine report writing lend themselves to project-based compensation more than open-ended analysis or expert witness services.

Former cardiac nurse Dr. Sandra Chen uses hybrid pricing strategies that match compensation methods to specific service types and client preferences. Her experience shows that different services require different pricing approaches for optimal results.

Sandra's medical record review services use hourly billing because document volume and complexity vary unpredictably between cases. Her expert witness services include retainer fees plus hourly billing for preparation and testimony time because clients need cost predictability for expert expenses.

Her standardized medical chronology services use project pricing because she's developed efficient processes that allow accurate cost estimation regardless of record volume. This pricing strategy provides competitive advantages while maintaining fair compensation for her expertise.

Retainer arrangements provide advance payment for future services while ensuring consultant availability during specific time periods. Retainers typically range from $2,500-15,000 depending on case complexity and expected service duration.

Value-based pricing considers case significance, damage amounts, and client budget capacity rather than simply calculating hourly rates multiplied by time estimates. High-value cases with substantial damage potential might justify premium pricing while smaller cases require fee adjustments.

Rush service premiums compensate for expedited work that requires schedule disruption, overtime hours, or deadline pressure that affects work quality or other client service. Premium rates typically add 25-50% to standard fees for urgent project completion.

Payment Terms and Collection Procedures

Payment scheduling options include advance payment requirements, progress billing during project completion, and final payment upon deliverable submission. Each approach offers different cash flow and risk management advantages depending on project scope and client reliability.

Advance payment requirements provide cash flow security while ensuring client commitment to project completion. However, some attorney clients prefer progress billing that matches payment obligations to work completion milestones.

Net payment terms typically range from net 15 to net 30 days after invoice submission, though some consultants require faster payment for cash flow management. Longer payment terms might be necessary for government clients or large law firms with established payment procedures.

Late payment penalties protect consultant cash flow while encouraging timely payment compliance. Typical penalties range from 1.5-2% per month on overdue balances, though state regulations might limit penalty amounts or assessment methods.

Collection procedures for overdue accounts should follow systematic approaches that preserve client relationships while protecting consultant interests. Early intervention often resolves payment delays without damaging professional relationships or requiring aggressive collection tactics.

The collection process typically begins with friendly payment reminders, escalates to formal demand letters, and might require collection agency services or legal action for persistent non-payment. Each escalation step increases collection costs while reducing relationship repair possibilities.

Former orthopedic nurse Margaret Davis learned collection importance through early career experiences with slow-paying attorney clients who created cash flow problems that threatened practice viability. Her experience led to systematic collection procedures that protect both relationships and finances.

Margaret's collection system includes payment reminder emails at 15 days past due, formal collection letters at 30 days, and collection agency referral at 60 days. The systematic approach resolves most payment delays without relationship damage while protecting against significant losses.

Her experience shows that most payment delays result from attorney cash flow problems or administrative oversights rather than payment refusal. Early intervention often resolves these problems without aggressive collection tactics that damage professional relationships.

Collection cost recovery provisions in service agreements allow consultants to recover attorney fees, collection agency costs, and administrative expenses for overdue account collection. These provisions reduce collection costs while encouraging voluntary payment compliance.

Credit application procedures for new clients help identify payment risks before beginning work on expensive projects. Credit applications might include bank references, trade references, and financial statement review for large consulting engagements.

Payment method preferences include traditional check payments, electronic transfers, and credit card processing that offer different advantages for cash flow management and payment security. Credit card processing provides immediate payment but includes transaction fees that reduce net compensation.

Tax Considerations and Deductions for LNCs

Business expense deductions provide significant tax advantages for legal nurse consulting practices that track expenses properly and maintain adequate documentation for IRS audit protection. Deductible expenses include office costs, professional development, equipment purchases, and travel expenses.

Home office deductions allow consultants working from home to deduct portion of housing costs including mortgage interest, property taxes, utilities, and maintenance expenses. The simplified home office deduction method allows $5 per square foot up to 300 square feet, while actual expense method might provide larger deductions for qualifying home offices.

Proper home office qualification requires exclusive business use of designated space for business purposes. Mixed-use areas like family rooms or kitchens generally don't qualify for home office deductions regardless of business activity frequency.

Professional development expenses include conference attendance, certification maintenance, continuing education, and professional association memberships that maintain or improve consulting skills. These investments often provide immediate tax deductions while building long-term practice value.

Equipment and technology deductions cover computer purchases, software licenses, office furniture, and communication equipment necessary for business operations. Section 179 depreciation rules allow immediate expense deduction for qualifying equipment purchases up to annual limits.

Former psychiatric nurse Dr. Robert Kim maximizes tax deductions through careful expense tracking and strategic business planning that reduces tax obligations while supporting practice growth. His systematic approach demonstrates effective tax management for consulting practices.

Robert's home office qualifies for actual expense deduction because he uses 200 square feet exclusively for business purposes. His home office deduction includes 15% of mortgage interest, property taxes, utilities, and home maintenance costs based on business space percentage.

His professional development expenses include AALNC membership, psychiatric nursing certification maintenance, legal nurse consulting conferences, and continuing education courses that maintain his specialized knowledge. These expenses provide immediate tax deductions while enhancing his expert witness qualifications.

Quarterly tax payments help consultants avoid year-end tax penalties and cash flow problems by spreading tax obligations throughout the year. Self-employed consultants typically must make quarterly estimated payments based on expected annual income.

Retirement plan contributions provide tax deductions while building long-term financial security through SEP-IRA, Solo 401k, or other self-employed retirement options. These plans often allow larger contributions than employee retirement plans while providing immediate tax benefits.

Business vehicle expenses can be deducted using either actual expense method or standard mileage rate for business travel to depositions, attorney meetings, and professional events. Proper documentation includes mileage logs, trip purposes, and expense receipts for audit protection.

Health insurance deductions for self-employed consultants allow deduction of health insurance premiums for themselves and family members as business expenses rather than itemized deductions subject to income limitations.

Building Your Business Foundation

The business structure and legal framework you establish today determines your practice's growth potential, risk exposure, and financial efficiency for years to come. These foundational decisions require careful analysis and professional guidance, but the investment in proper setup pays dividends through reduced liability, tax advantages, and professional credibility.

Your nursing background provides the clinical expertise that clients need, but business acumen separates successful consultants from those who struggle with administrative challenges. Master these business fundamentals to build a practice that supports both professional satisfaction and financial success.

Business Foundation Essentials for Long-Term Success

- LLC structure provides optimal liability protection and tax efficiency for most legal nurse consulting practices while maintaining operational flexibility

- Professional liability insurance coverage of $1-2 million protects against claims while meeting attorney client requirements for consulting engagement

- Written contracts with detailed scope, payment terms, and liability limitations prevent disputes while protecting consultant interests and client relationships

- Pricing strategies should match service types with hourly billing for variable work and project pricing for standardized deliverables

- Collection procedures require systematic approaches that preserve relationships while protecting cash flow through timely payment enforcement

- Tax planning through proper deductions and quarterly payments maximizes after-tax income while ensuring compliance with self-employment obligations

Chapter 11: Marketing That Actually Works for LNCs

Marketing legal nurse consulting services requires fundamentally different approaches than traditional healthcare career advancement—yet most nurses approach this challenge using networking methods that work for hospital positions but fail miserably with attorney clients. You need marketing strategies that build credibility with legal professionals who think differently, make decisions differently, and evaluate expertise using criteria that healthcare settings never taught you.

Successful legal nurse consultant marketing focuses on relationship building, credibility demonstration, and value proposition communication that resonates with attorney decision-making processes. The marketing methods that generate sustainable practices emphasize professional development, strategic networking, and systematic referral cultivation rather than traditional advertising approaches.

Attorney Networking Strategies That Build Relationships

Bar association participation provides direct access to attorney communities through continuing education events, committee involvement, and professional networking opportunities that allow relationship building over time. Local, state, and specialty bar associations offer different networking environments suited to various practice development goals.

Medical malpractice defense bar associations attract attorneys who regularly need legal nurse consulting services, making these organizations high-value networking targets. Plaintiff attorney associations also offer networking opportunities, though competition from other consultants might be more intense in these settings.

Speaking opportunities at bar association events position you as subject matter expert while demonstrating knowledge and communication skills that attorneys value in consultants. Educational presentations about medical topics, case study discussions, and panel participation create professional visibility with potential clients.

Successful speaking topics include healthcare trends affecting litigation, new medical technologies creating liability issues, and case studies that illustrate complex medical concepts. Focus on education rather than sales presentations to build credibility and professional relationships.

Former emergency nurse Dr. Jennifer Martinez built her practice through systematic bar association networking that began with attendance at medical malpractice seminars and evolved into regular speaking engagements about emergency medicine topics.

Jennifer's networking strategy started with monthly attendance at local medical malpractice defense bar meetings where she listened to attorney discussions about case challenges and expert witness needs. She introduced herself to attorneys after meetings, offered to answer medical questions, and provided business cards with her emergency medicine background.

Her consistent attendance led to informal consultation requests about emergency care standards and medication protocols. These conversations demonstrated her expertise while building relationships with attorneys who appreciated her practical knowledge and clear communication style.

Within six months, the bar association program chair invited Jennifer to present a program about emergency department care standards that could help attorneys understand emergency medicine litigation. Her presentation attracted 40 attorneys and generated several consulting requests from firms handling emergency medicine cases.

Professional relationship cultivation requires consistent follow-up, value-added communication, and long-term relationship investment that builds trust and familiarity with potential clients. Attorneys often work with consultants they know personally rather than selecting based solely on qualifications or competitive pricing.

Educational content sharing through newsletters, articles, and professional updates keeps your expertise visible to attorney networks while providing useful information that builds professional credibility. Regular communication maintains relationships during periods without active case work.

Committee participation in bar association activities provides leadership opportunities while building deeper relationships with attorney colleagues. Committee work demonstrates commitment to professional community while creating opportunities for extended interaction with potential clients.

Professional Association Leverage

American Association of Legal Nurse Consultants (AALNC) membership provides professional credibility, continuing education opportunities, and networking access to both legal nurse consultants and attorney members who support the organization's educational mission.

AALNC annual conferences attract hundreds of legal nurse consultants and attorney speakers who discuss case studies, practice development strategies, and industry trends that affect consulting opportunities. These events provide continuing education while enabling networking with potential referral sources.

Local chapter participation in AALNC affiliates offers regular networking opportunities with colleagues who might provide referrals, collaboration opportunities, or practice guidance. Chapter meetings often include attorney speakers who discuss consultant selection criteria and service expectations.

Volunteer leadership in AALNC chapters demonstrates professional commitment while building relationships with colleagues and attorney speakers. Newsletter editing, program planning, and educational committee participation create visibility within professional communities.

State nursing associations often include legal nurse consulting interest groups or continuing education programs that attract nurses considering career transitions. These organizations provide opportunities to mentor new consultants while building referral networks with nursing colleagues.

Specialty nursing associations related to your clinical background offer networking opportunities with nurses who might encounter legal consulting opportunities in their practice settings. ICU nurses, emergency department nurses, and other specialists often learn about cases requiring expert analysis.

Former surgical nurse Dr. Patricia Chen leveraged professional association membership to build a practice focusing on surgical malpractice and medical device litigation through systematic relationship building and leadership involvement.

Patricia's association strategy included AALNC membership with active local chapter participation, American Organization of Perioperative Registered Nurses (AORN) involvement, and state nursing association committee work that built relationships across multiple professional communities.

Her AALNC chapter leadership role as program coordinator allowed her to invite attorney speakers who discussed surgical malpractice trends and expert witness requirements. These relationships led to consulting opportunities with attorneys who appreciated her surgical expertise and professional presentation.

Her AORN involvement kept her current with surgical practice standards and device safety issues that became important in medical device litigation. The specialized knowledge from continued surgical nursing education enhanced her credibility with attorneys handling complex surgical cases.

Cross-referral networks develop naturally through professional association participation as colleagues learn about your practice areas and refer appropriate cases. Building referral relationships with consultants in different specialties creates mutual support systems that benefit all participants.

Continuing education credits from professional association events maintain nursing license requirements while providing networking opportunities and professional development that supports consulting practice growth.

Digital Marketing for Legal Professionals

Professional website development creates online presence that attorney clients expect from serious professional service providers. Legal websites require different content and presentation approaches than healthcare websites because attorney audiences have different information needs and decision-making criteria.

Website content should emphasize qualifications, case experience, and service offerings rather than general nursing expertise. Attorney visitors want to understand your specific legal consulting capabilities, not your clinical nursing background.

Search engine optimization for legal nurse consulting requires understanding attorney search patterns and keywords that potential clients use when seeking expert services. Local SEO optimization helps attorneys find consultants in their geographic area for cases requiring local expertise.

Professional website platforms like WordPress, Squarespace, or legal-specific website services provide templates and features designed for legal service providers. These platforms often include contact forms, service descriptions, and professional presentation features that serve attorney client needs.

LinkedIn professional networking offers powerful tools for building relationships with attorney clients through professional content sharing, connection building, and industry group participation. LinkedIn's legal professional network includes thousands of attorneys who use the platform for business development and expert identification.

LinkedIn content strategy should focus on educational posts about medical topics affecting litigation, case study discussions, and professional achievement sharing that demonstrates expertise without appearing sales-focused. Regular posting maintains visibility while building professional reputation.

Attorney-focused content creation includes blog posts, articles, and educational materials that address legal issues from medical perspectives. Content topics might include healthcare trends affecting litigation, medical technology developments, and case studies that illustrate expert analysis approaches.

Former critical care nurse Dr. Michael Rodriguez built his practice through strategic digital marketing that combined professional website development with LinkedIn networking and content creation focused on critical care litigation topics.

Michael's website emphasized his ICU experience, expert witness qualifications, and case results rather than general nursing background. The site included detailed service descriptions, fee information, and client testimonials that helped attorneys understand his capabilities.

His LinkedIn strategy included regular posts about critical care topics affecting litigation, commentary on healthcare news with legal implications, and case study discussions that demonstrated his analytical approach. These posts generated connection requests from attorneys and referrals from colleagues.

The combined digital marketing approach created online visibility that attracted inquiries from attorneys handling critical care cases. His professional online presence supported his networking efforts while providing credibility verification for potential clients.

Online review management helps maintain positive professional reputation through client testimonials and professional references that attorney clients can verify. Legal professionals often research expert consultants thoroughly before engagement, making online reputation management essential.

Email marketing systems for professional communication help maintain relationships with attorney clients through regular updates, educational content, and case availability notifications. Professional email platforms provide tracking and automation features that support systematic client communication.

Referral Systems and Client Retention

Systematic referral cultivation requires identifying referral sources, maintaining regular contact, and providing value that encourages continued referrals over time. Successful referral systems combine current client satisfaction with new relationship development for sustainable practice growth.

Current client satisfaction provides the foundation for referral generation because satisfied attorneys recommend trusted consultants to colleagues handling similar cases. Excellent service delivery, timely communication, and professional reliability create client advocates who generate organic referrals.

Professional excellence standards in every client interaction build reputation for reliability and expertise that encourages repeat business and referral generation. Consistent high-quality service delivery creates client confidence that supports long-term relationship development.

Follow-up procedures after case completion maintain relationships during periods without active work while creating opportunities for future engagement. Regular contact with past clients keeps your services visible for new case opportunities.

Value-added services like educational presentations, article sharing, and consultation availability beyond formal case work build relationship depth while demonstrating ongoing commitment to client success. These activities create client loyalty that supports referral generation.

Former obstetric nurse Dr. Linda Foster developed successful referral systems through systematic client relationship management and professional excellence that generated sustainable practice growth without extensive marketing investment.

Linda's client retention strategy included detailed case follow-up procedures that maintained contact with attorneys after case completion. She sent thank-you notes, requested feedback, and provided updates about her continuing education and professional development activities.

Her value-added services included quarterly newsletters with obstetric litigation updates, offer to answer quick questions without billing, and availability for emergency consultations that demonstrated commitment to client success beyond formal case work.

The systematic approach generated referrals from satisfied clients who recommended Linda to colleagues handling obstetric cases. Her reputation for reliability and expertise created demand that exceeded her capacity within three years of practice establishment.

Referral tracking systems help identify successful referral sources and relationship cultivation opportunities through systematic monitoring of inquiry sources and conversion rates. Understanding referral patterns guides marketing investment and relationship development priorities.

Professional networking databases maintain contact information, relationship history, and follow-up schedules for potential referral sources. CRM systems designed for professional services help organize relationship management activities and communication scheduling.

Professional Branding and Credibility Building

Professional brand development creates consistent identity and messaging that communicates expertise, reliability, and value proposition to attorney clients. Effective branding differentiates your services while building recognition and trust with potential clients.

Brand elements include professional logo design, consistent color schemes, standardized communication templates, and messaging that emphasizes your unique qualifications and service approach. Professional branding creates credibility while supporting marketing effectiveness.

Credibility demonstration through published articles, speaking engagements, and professional recognition builds expert reputation that attorney clients value when selecting consultants. Published thought leadership creates evidence of expertise that supports marketing efforts.

Writing opportunities include legal nursing journals, bar association publications, and professional newsletters that reach attorney audiences. Article topics should address medical issues affecting litigation while demonstrating analytical thinking and communication skills.

Professional photography and materials create polished presentation that meets attorney expectations for professional service providers. High-quality headshots, business cards, and marketing materials reflect professional standards while building credibility.

Case study development showcases successful consulting engagements while demonstrating analytical approach and value delivery to potential clients. Case studies should focus on problem-solving methodology rather than specific case details to maintain confidentiality.

Professional awards and recognition from nursing and legal communities provide third-party validation of expertise and professional excellence. Award applications and professional recognition opportunities create credibility while building professional visibility.

Former pediatric nurse Dr. Susan Taylor built professional brand through systematic credibility development that included publication, speaking, and professional recognition activities that established her as pediatric litigation expert.

Susan's branding strategy included professional website development with pediatric expertise emphasis, published articles about child abuse investigation and pediatric emergency care standards, and speaking engagements at medical and legal conferences.

Her professional recognition included AALNC chapter president appointment, state nursing association award for professional excellence, and invitation to serve on hospital medical staff committee addressing pediatric emergency care protocols.

The systematic branding effort created professional recognition that generated referrals from attorneys, pediatricians, and social service agencies handling child abuse and medical malpractice cases involving pediatric patients.

The 18 Common Marketing Mistakes to Avoid

Mistake 1: Generic marketing materials that fail to address attorney-specific needs and decision-making criteria. Healthcare marketing approaches don't translate effectively to legal professional audiences who have different priorities and evaluation methods.

Mistake 2: Networking without follow-up systems that fail to convert initial contacts into ongoing relationships. Meeting attorneys at events without systematic follow-up wastes networking investment and relationship opportunities.

Mistake 3: Inadequate professional presentation including poor-quality business cards, unprofessional email addresses, and casual communication that undermines credibility with legal professional audiences.

Mistake 4: Overemphasis on nursing credentials without sufficient focus on legal consulting capabilities and case experience. Attorneys need consultants who understand legal requirements, not just clinical medicine.

Mistake 5: Inconsistent marketing efforts that create sporadic visibility without sustained relationship building or professional recognition development. Effective marketing requires consistent long-term investment rather than occasional activities.

Mistake 6: Failure to understand attorney decision-making processes and selection criteria for expert consultants. Attorneys evaluate consultants differently than healthcare employers, requiring different marketing approaches.

Mistake 7: Inadequate online presence including outdated websites, minimal LinkedIn profiles, and lack of professional digital visibility that attorney clients expect from serious consultants.

Mistake 8: Poor pricing communication that fails to provide clear fee information or creates confusion about service costs. Attorneys need cost predictability for budget planning and client communication.

Mistake 9: Neglecting referral cultivation by failing to maintain relationships with past clients and potential referral sources. Referrals generate the most cost-effective new business for consulting practices.

Mistake 10: Inappropriate professional boundaries including social media connection with clients, personal information sharing, and casual communication that undermines professional credibility.

Mistake 11: Insufficient continuing education that fails to maintain current knowledge about practice standards and legal developments affecting consulting areas. Outdated knowledge undermines expert credibility.

Mistake 12: Poor time management for marketing activities that results in sporadic efforts without sustained relationship building or professional development investment.

Mistake 13: Inadequate case portfolio development that fails to document successful consulting experiences and professional achievements that support marketing efforts.

Mistake 14: Weak professional associations participation that misses networking opportunities and professional development resources available through membership organizations.

Mistake 15: Failure to differentiate services from competitors through specialized expertise, unique qualifications, or distinctive service approaches that create competitive advantages.

Mistake 16: Inadequate client feedback systems that miss opportunities to improve service delivery and build client satisfaction that generates referrals and repeat business.

Mistake 17: Poor professional communication including delayed response times, unclear correspondence, and inadequate documentation that damages client relationships and professional reputation.

Mistake 18: Insufficient business development planning that lacks systematic approach to practice growth, relationship cultivation, and professional recognition development over time.

Creating Marketing Momentum

Effective marketing for legal nurse consulting requires systematic relationship building, professional credibility development, and consistent value delivery that builds trust with attorney clients over time. The most successful consultants combine networking excellence with professional development and service quality that creates sustainable competitive advantages.

Your clinical expertise provides the foundation, but marketing skills determine how effectively you can connect that expertise with attorney clients who need your services. Invest in relationship building and professional development to create marketing momentum that supports long-term practice success.

Marketing Excellence Framework for Sustainable Growth

- Attorney networking through bar associations and speaking opportunities builds relationships with potential clients who regularly need consulting services

- Professional association participation provides credibility, continuing education, and networking opportunities that support practice development and referral generation

- Digital marketing including professional websites and LinkedIn networking creates online visibility that attorney clients expect from serious consultants

- Referral systems and client retention through systematic relationship management generate the most cost-effective new business for consulting practices

- Professional branding and credibility building through publication and recognition activities establish expert reputation that supports marketing effectiveness

- Common marketing mistakes include generic materials, poor follow-up, inadequate presentation, and insufficient relationship cultivation that undermine practice development

Chapter 12: Client Acquisition and Relationship Management

Building a sustainable legal nurse consulting practice requires more than clinical expertise and professional credentials—you need systematic approaches to identifying ideal clients, converting initial contacts into long-term relationships, and expanding services within existing attorney partnerships. Most consultants struggle with client acquisition because they approach attorneys using networking methods that work for healthcare colleagues but fail with legal professionals who evaluate service providers differently.

Successful client acquisition combines targeted prospecting with relationship development strategies that demonstrate value while building trust over time. The most profitable consulting practices focus on developing deep relationships with select attorney clients rather than pursuing numerous superficial contacts that generate sporadic project work.

Identifying Ideal Attorney Clients

Practice area alignment represents the most critical factor in identifying attorney clients who can provide consistent, high-value consulting opportunities. Attorneys specializing in medical malpractice, personal injury, products liability, and workers' compensation regularly need medical expertise for case development and litigation support.

Large law firms handling complex litigation often need multiple consultants with different specializations, creating opportunities for ongoing relationships that generate substantial revenue over time. Small firms specializing in medical cases might provide fewer individual projects but offer closer working relationships and faster decision-making processes.

Geographic considerations affect client development strategies because local attorneys prefer consultants familiar with regional healthcare systems, practice standards, and expert witness pools. However, complex cases often justify consultant travel, and remote work capabilities expand geographic market access significantly.

Client size affects project characteristics and payment reliability in predictable patterns. Large firms typically offer bigger projects with higher fees but slower payment cycles and more complex approval processes. Small firms might provide faster turnaround and personal relationships but smaller project scope and budget constraints.

Specialization matching between your clinical background and attorney practice areas creates competitive advantages that generic consultants cannot replicate. Emergency medicine experience provides unique qualifications for trauma litigation, while surgical background supports medical device and procedure-related cases.

Former cardiac surgery nurse Dr. Patricia Thompson identified ideal clients through systematic market research that analyzed local attorney practices, case types, and consultant utilization patterns to target the most promising opportunities.

Patricia's market analysis revealed three large firms specializing in medical device litigation with national client bases requiring extensive cardiac surgery expertise. She also identified five smaller firms handling cardiac malpractice cases with regular expert witness needs.

Her research included reviewing firm websites, case results, and news articles about major settlements to understand their practice patterns and consultant requirements. This analysis helped her tailor approach strategies to each firm's specific needs and decision-making processes.

The targeted approach generated initial consultations with decision-makers who appreciated her preparation and understanding of their practice requirements. Her focused strategy proved more effective than broad networking approaches that consumed more time while generating fewer qualified opportunities.

Financial stability assessment helps identify attorney clients who can pay consulting fees promptly and sustain long-term working relationships. Firms with consistent case flow and established payment systems provide more reliable income than those handling occasional cases or experiencing financial difficulties.

Case volume analysis determines potential consulting opportunity frequency and revenue sustainability from different attorney relationships. Firms handling multiple medical cases monthly offer more stable income potential than those with sporadic case loads.

Decision-maker identification within law firms helps focus relationship development efforts on attorneys who can authorize consulting engagements rather than junior associates or support staff who cannot make hiring decisions.

Initial Consultation Strategies

Preparation protocols for attorney meetings require research about their practice areas, recent cases, and consultant utilization patterns to demonstrate professional preparation and genuine interest in their business needs. Attorneys appreciate consultants who understand their practice challenges and case requirements.

Initial consultation goals include demonstrating expertise, understanding client needs, explaining service capabilities, and establishing professional credibility that supports future engagement. These meetings often determine if attorneys will consider you for consulting opportunities.

Consultation structure should include introduction and background sharing, practice area discussion, case examples that demonstrate analytical approach, service explanation with fee information, and next steps identification for potential engagement.

Value demonstration during consultations requires sharing specific examples of how your expertise has helped similar clients achieve case success, identify liability issues, or develop expert witness strategies. Case studies provide concrete evidence of value delivery.

Question preparation helps guide consultations toward productive discussions about attorney needs, current consultant relationships, and opportunities for future collaboration. Thoughtful questions demonstrate professional interest while gathering information needed for relationship development.

Former obstetric nurse Dr. Jennifer Martinez developed effective consultation strategies through systematic preparation and structured presentations that consistently converted initial meetings into consulting engagements.

Jennifer's consultation preparation included reviewing attorney websites, researching recent case results, and identifying potential challenges in their practice areas that her obstetric expertise could address effectively.

Her consultation presentations included three case studies showing how her analysis identified care standard violations, contributed to successful settlements, and provided expert witness testimony that helped attorneys achieve favorable outcomes.

The structured approach demonstrated her analytical capabilities while showing attorneys how her services could benefit their practice. Her preparation and professionalism differentiated her from competitors who approached consultations casually.

Professional presentation during consultations includes appropriate dress, punctual arrival, organized materials, and confident communication that builds credibility with attorney audiences accustomed to high professional standards.

Follow-up procedures after consultations maintain momentum while providing additional information that supports engagement decisions. Systematic follow-up often determines if initial contacts develop into working relationships.

Objection handling for common attorney concerns about consultant costs, qualifications, or service approaches requires prepared responses that address issues while maintaining positive relationship development.

Proposal Writing That Wins Cases

Proposal structure for legal nurse consulting services requires clear problem identification, solution approach explanation, deliverable specification, timeline establishment, and cost estimation that helps attorneys make informed engagement decisions.

Winning proposals demonstrate understanding of attorney needs while explaining how your specific expertise addresses their case challenges effectively. Generic proposals rarely generate engagement because they fail to connect consultant capabilities with client requirements.

Scope definition prevents misunderstandings about deliverable requirements while establishing clear boundaries for consulting engagement. Detailed scope statements protect both consultants and clients from unrealistic expectations or project expansion without additional compensation.

Service proposals should include background review requirements, analysis methodology, deliverable formats, communication protocols, and timeline expectations that guide project completion. Clear expectations prevent disputes while ensuring client satisfaction.

Value proposition articulation explains how your consulting services provide benefits that justify engagement costs through improved case outcomes, expert witness quality, or litigation efficiency. Attorneys need clear benefit explanations to justify consultant expenses.

Competitive differentiation in proposals highlights unique qualifications, specialized experience, or distinctive approaches that separate your services from other available consultants. Differentiation helps attorneys understand why they should select your services over alternatives.

Former emergency medicine nurse Dr. Michael Rodriguez developed proposal writing skills that consistently won consulting engagements through clear value demonstration and competitive differentiation strategies.

Michael's proposals for emergency medicine cases emphasized his 15-year emergency department experience, board certification in emergency nursing, and expert witness track record with successful testimony in similar cases.

His proposals included specific case examples showing how his analysis identified care standard violations, timeline development that revealed critical decision points, and expert opinions that contributed to favorable case outcomes for attorney clients.

The detailed proposals demonstrated his analytical approach while showing attorneys how his services would specifically benefit their cases. His systematic proposal writing generated engagement rates exceeding 75% for qualified opportunities.

Cost-benefit analysis in proposals helps attorneys understand return on investment for consulting services through case value improvement, settlement probability enhancement, or litigation cost reduction.

Risk assessment sections address potential challenges or limitations that might affect consulting outcomes while demonstrating professional honesty and realistic expectation setting.

Implementation planning provides detailed project timelines, milestone identification, and communication schedules that help attorneys plan case development activities around consulting deliverables.

Project Management and Communication Systems

Project organization for complex consulting engagements requires systematic approaches that track multiple tasks, deadlines, and deliverables while maintaining quality standards and client communication throughout project completion.

Professional project management tools help organize case materials, track progress, and communicate status to attorney clients who need regular updates about consulting work completion. These systems prevent missed deadlines while ensuring quality deliverable preparation.

Communication protocols establish regular contact schedules, preferred communication methods, and response time expectations that maintain attorney satisfaction while managing consultant workload efficiently.

Attorney clients typically prefer email communication with formal documentation of important discussions and decisions. Phone conversations should be followed by email summaries that confirm key points and action items.

Status reporting provides regular updates about project progress, challenges encountered, and completion timeline modifications that help attorneys plan case development activities around consulting deliverables.

Quality assurance procedures ensure deliverable accuracy and completeness before submission to attorney clients. Systematic quality checks prevent errors that could damage consultant credibility or client relationships.

Former surgical nurse Dr. Sandra Chen developed project management systems that enabled simultaneous handling of multiple complex cases while maintaining quality standards and client satisfaction across all engagements.

Sandra's project management approach included digital case files with organized document storage, task tracking systems with deadline alerts, and standardized communication templates that ensured consistent client updates.

Her quality assurance procedures included peer review for complex analyses, accuracy verification for medical facts and timeline, and professional editing for all written deliverables before client submission.

The systematic approach enabled Sandra to handle 15-20 active cases simultaneously while maintaining quality standards that generated client satisfaction and referral opportunities for practice growth.

Time management for multiple concurrent projects requires prioritization systems that balance urgent deadlines with long-term project requirements while maintaining quality standards across all engagements.

Technology integration including case management software, communication platforms, and collaboration tools helps streamline project administration while improving client service quality and consultant efficiency.

Escalation procedures for project challenges help address problems quickly while maintaining client relationships and project completion timelines.

Building Long-Term Partnerships

Relationship development beyond individual projects requires ongoing communication, value delivery, and professional support that creates attorney loyalty and preference for your consulting services over competitor alternatives.

Long-term partnerships provide practice stability through predictable case flow, premium pricing acceptance, and referral generation that reduces marketing investment while increasing revenue sustainability.

Trust building through consistent quality delivery, reliable communication, and professional integrity creates attorney confidence that supports long-term relationship development and consulting engagement expansion.

Professional development sharing with attorney clients including continuing education updates, certification achievements, and specialized training completion demonstrates ongoing expertise development while maintaining relationship visibility.

Strategic consultation beyond formal case work provides value-added services that build relationship depth while demonstrating consulting expertise and professional commitment to client success.

Former critical care nurse Dr. Robert Kim built long-term partnerships through systematic relationship development that generated sustainable practice growth with premium compensation and minimal marketing investment.

Robert's partnership development included quarterly client communications with practice updates, continuing education achievements, and industry trend analysis that affected critical care litigation.

His value-added services included availability for quick consultation questions, emergency case review for urgent deadlines, and educational presentations about critical care topics for attorney continuing education programs.

The systematic partnership approach generated client loyalty that resulted in exclusive consulting relationships with three major firms and referral streams that exceeded his practice capacity within five years.

Client feedback systems help identify service improvement opportunities while demonstrating professional commitment to client satisfaction and relationship development.

Service expansion opportunities within existing relationships provide revenue growth through additional service offerings that leverage established trust and proven performance with attorney clients.

Exclusive relationship agreements with select attorney clients provide income predictability while ensuring consultant availability for important cases and urgent consulting needs.

Expanding Services Within Existing Relationships

Service portfolio development beyond basic consulting includes expert witness services, staff training, case strategy development, and specialized analysis that increase engagement value while building revenue within existing relationships.

Cross-selling strategies for related services help maximize revenue from satisfied clients who trust your expertise and service quality. Existing relationships provide the best opportunities for service expansion because trust and performance history support new service acceptance.

Upselling approaches for enhanced service levels include expedited delivery, additional analysis depth, or premium support options that provide increased value while generating higher compensation from existing engagements.

Training and education services for attorney staff about medical topics, case analysis approaches, or expert witness preparation provide additional revenue while building relationship depth and client dependency.

Retainer arrangements for ongoing availability provide stable income while ensuring client access to consulting services for urgent needs or regular case review requirements.

Former pediatric nurse Dr. Lisa Park expanded services within existing relationships through systematic portfolio development that increased per-client revenue while building competitive advantages for long-term practice sustainability.

Lisa's service expansion began with basic consulting services and evolved to include expert witness testimony, attorney staff training about pediatric medicine, and ongoing case strategy consultation for complex pediatric litigation.

Her training programs for attorney staff covered pediatric development, injury patterns, and medical terminology that helped legal teams better understand pediatric cases and expert witness testimony.

The expanded services generated 60% revenue increase from existing clients while creating competitive barriers that prevented client migration to other consultants offering only basic services.

Partnership agreements with attorney clients for complex cases or ongoing legal needs provide revenue stability while ensuring consultant involvement in significant litigation opportunities.

Collaborative relationship development includes joint case strategy sessions, expert witness preparation coordination, and litigation support that positions consultants as essential team members rather than external service providers.

Performance measurement for service expansion initiatives helps identify successful approaches while optimizing resource allocation for maximum revenue growth and client satisfaction within existing relationships.

Transforming Contacts Into Partnerships

Client acquisition and relationship management represent core business skills that determine consulting practice success more than clinical expertise or professional credentials. The most successful legal nurse consultants excel at identifying ideal clients, converting opportunities into engagements, and building long-term partnerships that provide sustainable revenue growth.

Your nursing background provides the clinical foundation, but business development skills determine how effectively you can build relationships with attorney clients who need your expertise. Master these client development fundamentals to create a practice that generates both professional satisfaction and financial success.

Client Development Mastery for Sustainable Success

- Ideal client identification requires practice area alignment, geographic considerations, and specialization matching that creates competitive advantages over generic consultants

- Initial consultation strategies need systematic preparation and structured presentations that demonstrate expertise while understanding attorney needs and decision-making processes

- Proposal writing must include clear value propositions, competitive differentiation, and detailed scope definitions that help attorneys make informed engagement decisions

- Project management systems enable multiple concurrent cases while maintaining quality standards and client satisfaction through organized communication and systematic delivery

- Long-term partnership building requires ongoing relationship development, trust creation, and value-added services that generate client loyalty and sustainable revenue growth

- Service expansion within existing relationships provides the most cost-effective revenue growth through cross-selling, upselling, and portfolio development that leverages established trust

Chapter 13: Quality Assurance and Risk Management

Professional excellence in legal nurse consulting requires more than clinical expertise—it demands systematic quality assurance processes that prevent errors, manage risks, and maintain the standards that separate credible consultants from those who damage the profession's reputation. Your analysis might influence million-dollar legal decisions, yet many consultants operate without the quality control systems that protect both clients and professional standing.

The difference between competent analysis and professional excellence lies in the systematic approaches you develop to catch errors, verify accuracy, and maintain objectivity under pressure. These quality assurance frameworks become your professional insurance policy, protecting against the costly mistakes that can destroy consulting careers and damage client relationships permanently.

Error Prevention Systems and Double-Checking Protocols

Systematic review protocols provide the foundation for error prevention by establishing consistent analytical processes that reduce oversight risks and ensure thorough case evaluation. These protocols should address every phase of case analysis from initial record organization through final report preparation.

The three-phase verification system offers reliable error detection across different analytical stages. Phase one involves initial record review with preliminary timeline development and issue identification. Phase two includes detailed analysis with literature research and opinion formation. Phase three encompasses final review with accuracy verification and quality checking before client delivery.

Document verification procedures ensure accuracy of factual information that forms the foundation of your analysis. Medical record transcription errors, date mistakes, and medication dosage inaccuracies can undermine entire case analyses if not detected and corrected during systematic review processes.

Create verification checklists that address common error categories including chronological accuracy, medical terminology consistency, medication dosage verification, and timeline coordination across multiple record sources. These checklists provide systematic approaches to accuracy verification that prevent embarrassing mistakes.

Former ICU nurse Dr. Patricia Martinez learned the importance of systematic error prevention when a medication dosage transcription error in her analysis nearly derailed a $2 million malpractice case and damaged her relationship with a major law firm client.

Patricia's analysis of a post-operative infection case included detailed medication administration review showing appropriate antibiotic therapy according to hospital protocols. However, her transcription error recorded antibiotic dosage as 500 mg when medical records clearly showed 50 mg—a ten-fold error that completely changed the clinical significance.

The opposing expert witness identified Patricia's transcription error during cross-examination, using it to challenge her attention to detail and overall analysis credibility. Although the error didn't affect her ultimate conclusions about care standard violations, it damaged her professional reputation and required extensive damage control.

The experience led Patricia to develop systematic verification protocols including independent review of all factual data, cross-checking of medication information against multiple record sources, and peer review for complex cases requiring detailed pharmaceutical analysis.

Literature verification systems ensure accuracy of medical information and care standards that support your analysis and opinions. Outdated guidelines, misquoted studies, or inaccurate medical facts can destroy consultant credibility when discovered by opposing experts.

Professional medical databases including PubMed, Cochrane Reviews, and specialty organization websites provide authoritative sources for current care standards and clinical guidelines. Avoid general internet sources or outdated textbooks that might contain inaccurate or obsolete information.

Peer consultation networks provide independent verification for complex cases requiring specialized knowledge beyond your expertise. Building relationships with consultants in different specialties creates resource networks for challenging analytical questions.

Professional Boundaries and Ethical Considerations

Scope of practice limitations require understanding the boundaries between nursing knowledge and areas requiring other professional expertise. Legal nurse consultants must recognize when cases require physician, pharmacist, or other specialized knowledge that exceeds nursing scope.

Medical diagnosis and treatment recommendations fall outside nursing scope of practice, even in consulting contexts. Your analysis should focus on nursing care standards, patient safety issues, and healthcare delivery problems rather than medical diagnosis or treatment appropriateness.

Objectivity maintenance becomes challenging when personal beliefs, previous experiences, or case emotional content affects professional judgment. Systematic approaches to bias recognition and objectivity preservation protect analytical accuracy and professional credibility.

Document your analytical reasoning process to identify potential bias sources and ensure conclusions follow from evidence rather than personal preferences. This systematic approach provides protection against unconscious bias that might compromise analysis quality.

Confidentiality obligations extend beyond HIPAA requirements to include attorney work product protection and case strategy confidentiality. Legal nurse consultants must understand complex confidentiality requirements that differ from traditional healthcare settings.

Former emergency nurse Dr. Michael Rodriguez faced ethical challenges when asked to review a case involving a colleague from his previous hospital employment. The personal relationship created potential bias that required careful boundary management.

Michael's systematic approach included disclosure of the relationship to the attorney client, documentation of potential bias sources, and peer consultation to verify analytical objectivity. His transparent handling preserved both professional relationships and analytical credibility.

The case involved allegations of delayed stroke recognition in the emergency department where Michael had previously worked. His personal knowledge of departmental protocols and staff capabilities could have influenced his analysis inappropriately.

Michael's solution included focusing analysis on documented care standards rather than personal knowledge of individual capabilities, using only information available in medical records, and obtaining peer review from consultants without hospital connection.

Conflict of interest identification requires systematic evaluation of personal, professional, and financial relationships that might compromise analytical objectivity. These conflicts can be subtle but devastating if discovered during litigation.

Professional boundary maintenance with attorney clients includes appropriate communication styles, service scope limitations, and relationship management that preserves professional credibility while building effective working partnerships.

Ethical consultation resources including professional organizations and ethical guidelines provide guidance for complex situations requiring professional judgment about appropriate consultant behavior.

Conflict of Interest Identification and Management

Financial conflict assessment examines potential monetary benefits that might influence analytical conclusions including stock ownership in defendant companies, consulting relationships with involved parties, or financial interests in case outcomes.

Healthcare consultants often own stock in pharmaceutical companies, medical device manufacturers, or healthcare corporations that might be involved in litigation. These financial interests create potential conflicts that require disclosure or case declination.

Professional relationship conflicts arise when consultants have current or previous working relationships with involved healthcare providers, institutions, or organizations that might affect analytical objectivity.

Previous employment at defendant institutions, consulting relationships with involved parties, or professional friendships with key witnesses create conflicts that require careful evaluation and appropriate management or case declination.

Personal relationship conflicts include family connections, social relationships, or personal experiences that might compromise analytical objectivity or create appearance of bias problems.

Expert witness conflicts occur when consultants have previous testimony history in related cases or existing relationships with opposing experts that might affect current case analysis or testimony credibility.

Former surgical nurse Dr. Jennifer Williams encountered complex conflict issues when asked to review a case involving medical device failure from a manufacturer where her spouse worked as an engineer.

Jennifer's conflict analysis revealed that her spouse's employment created potential bias appearance even though he worked in a different division unrelated to the problematic device. The financial benefit from her husband's employment could appear to influence her analysis.

Her conflict management approach included full disclosure to the attorney client, documentation of the employment relationship and its limitations, and offer to decline the case if the attorney preferred avoiding any appearance of bias.

The attorney appreciated Jennifer's transparency and chose to engage her services based on her unique surgical expertise, with full understanding of the potential conflict. Jennifer's careful documentation protected both parties from later conflict challenges.

Conflict disclosure procedures require systematic documentation of potential conflicts and appropriate communication with attorney clients about conflict implications and management strategies.

Conflict monitoring systems help track ongoing conflicts as cases develop and new information emerges that might create previously unknown conflict situations.

Case declination criteria establish clear guidelines for situations requiring case refusal due to unmanageable conflicts that compromise analytical objectivity or professional credibility.

Documentation and Record-Keeping Requirements

Case file organization systems ensure systematic storage and retrieval of all materials related to consulting engagements including contracts, records, correspondence, research materials, and deliverables.

Professional case management requires organized documentation that supports quality analysis while protecting against claims of inadequate work or missing materials. These systems become essential during litigation when opposing counsel might question consultant preparation and analysis methods.

Time tracking documentation provides detailed records of all activities related to consulting engagements including record review, research, analysis, consultation, and communication time for billing accuracy and professional credibility.

Accurate time records protect against billing disputes while demonstrating thorough case preparation and analysis. These records often become evidence of consultant preparation quality during cross-examination or billing challenge situations.

Research documentation includes systematic records of literature sources, database searches, and reference materials that support analytical conclusions and expert opinions.

Opposing experts often challenge consultant research methods and source quality during cross-examination. Detailed research documentation demonstrates thorough preparation while supporting analytical credibility and opinion foundation.

Former pediatric nurse Dr. Sandra Chen developed systematic documentation protocols after learning from early career challenges with inadequate record-keeping that created professional and legal problems.

Sandra's documentation system includes electronic case files with standardized folder structures, comprehensive time tracking with detailed activity descriptions, and research logs documenting all literature sources and database searches.

Her systematic approach proved valuable when opposing counsel challenged her research methods during deposition in a pediatric malpractice case. Her detailed documentation demonstrated thorough literature review and appropriate research methodology.

The opposing attorney's attempt to portray her as inadequately prepared backfired when Sandra's research documentation showed extensive preparation exceeding opposing expert efforts. Her systematic approach strengthened her credibility while protecting against unfair challenges.

Communication documentation requires systematic records of all client interactions including meeting notes, email correspondence, and phone conversation summaries that protect against misunderstandings or disputed instructions.

Quality assurance documentation includes records of verification procedures, peer consultations, and accuracy checking processes that demonstrate systematic quality control and professional excellence.

Retention requirements for case documentation vary by jurisdiction and contract requirements but typically require storage for multiple years after case completion to support potential appeals or related litigation.

Professional Development and Continuing Education

Continuing education requirements for legal nurse consultants include nursing license maintenance, professional certification updates, and specialized training that maintains current knowledge about practice standards and legal developments.

Systematic professional development planning ensures continuous knowledge updates while building credentials that support expert witness qualification and professional credibility with attorney clients.

Specialty knowledge maintenance requires ongoing education about specific clinical areas relevant to your consulting practice including new treatments, revised guidelines, and emerging research that affects care standards.

Legal nurse consultants must stay current with both clinical developments and legal trends that affect consulting practice. This dual requirement demands systematic educational planning and resource allocation.

Legal education components help consultants understand litigation processes, legal requirements, and courtroom procedures that affect consulting effectiveness and expert witness performance.

Understanding legal concepts, evidence rules, and courtroom procedures improves consultant effectiveness while building credibility with attorney clients who appreciate legal sophistication.

Former emergency medicine nurse Dr. Robert Kim developed systematic professional development programs that maintained both clinical currency and legal sophistication required for effective consulting practice.

Robert's educational plan included annual emergency medicine conferences, legal nurse consulting continuing education, courtroom skills training, and specialized programs about emerging technologies affecting emergency care.

His systematic approach included budget allocation for professional development, educational goal setting with measurable objectives, and performance tracking that demonstrated knowledge acquisition and application.

The investment in professional development paid dividends through enhanced expert witness qualifications, improved case analysis capabilities, and attorney client recognition of his professional sophistication and current knowledge.

Certification maintenance for nursing licenses and professional credentials requires systematic tracking of educational requirements, renewal deadlines, and compliance documentation.

Professional reading programs help maintain current knowledge through systematic review of professional journals, legal publications, and specialty literature relevant to consulting practice areas.

Conference attendance strategies maximize educational value while building professional networks that support practice development and knowledge acquisition.

Peer Review and Mentorship Opportunities

Peer consultation networks provide independent verification for complex cases, quality assurance for challenging analyses, and professional support for difficult consulting situations.

Building relationships with experienced consultants in similar and complementary specialties creates resource networks for professional development and quality improvement initiatives.

Formal peer review programs through professional organizations offer systematic quality assessment and improvement feedback that helps consultants identify strengths and development opportunities.

These programs provide independent evaluation of analytical methods, report quality, and professional practices that support continuous improvement and credibility building.

Mentorship relationships with experienced legal nurse consultants provide guidance for practice development, professional challenges, and career advancement opportunities.

Effective mentorship includes both formal programs through professional organizations and informal relationships with successful consultants willing to share knowledge and experience.

Quality improvement initiatives through peer collaboration help identify best practices, develop improved analytical methods, and build professional standards that benefit the entire consulting community.

Former cardiac surgery nurse Dr. Lisa Park built peer review networks that improved her practice quality while providing professional support during challenging cases and career development decisions.

Lisa's peer network included consultants in cardiac surgery, cardiology, and related specialties who provided consultation for complex cases and quality review for challenging analyses.

Her formal mentorship relationship with an experienced expert witness helped her develop courtroom skills, understand legal requirements, and build confidence for testimony in high-stakes litigation.

The peer support network proved invaluable when Lisa faced aggressive cross-examination in a complex cardiac device case. Her mentor's guidance and peer consultation helped her prepare effectively and maintain credibility under pressure.

Professional organization involvement provides access to peer networks, quality improvement resources, and mentorship opportunities that support practice development and professional growth.

Knowledge sharing activities including conference presentations, article writing, and educational program development contribute to professional community while building personal recognition and credibility.

Collaborative quality initiatives with other consultants help develop industry standards, improve analytical methods, and address professional challenges that affect consulting effectiveness.

Professional Standards in Practice

Quality assurance and risk management separate professional legal nurse consultants from those who damage the profession through careless analysis and unprofessional conduct. The systematic approaches outlined here provide frameworks for maintaining excellence while managing the risks inherent in complex consulting practice.

Your commitment to quality assurance affects not only your individual success but also the reputation and credibility of legal nurse consulting as a profession. Professional excellence requires ongoing attention to quality systems, ethical practices, and continuous improvement that builds lasting success.

Quality Excellence Framework for Professional Success

- Error prevention systems including systematic review protocols and verification procedures protect against costly mistakes that damage professional credibility and client relationships

- Professional boundaries and ethical considerations require understanding scope limitations, maintaining objectivity, and managing confidentiality obligations appropriately

- Conflict of interest identification and management prevent bias appearance while protecting analytical credibility through systematic disclosure and documentation procedures

- Documentation and record-keeping systems provide professional protection while demonstrating thorough preparation and systematic analytical approaches

- Professional development and continuing education maintain current knowledge while building credentials that support expert witness qualification and client confidence

- Peer review and mentorship opportunities improve practice quality while providing professional support for challenging cases and career development decisions

Chapter 14: Scaling Your LNC Practice

The transformation from individual consultant to practice leader requires fundamentally different skills than those that built your initial success—yet most legal nurse consultants approach growth using the same methods that worked for solo practice but fail catastrophically when applied to team management and business scaling. You need systematic approaches to delegation, quality control, and business development that maintain service excellence while increasing capacity and revenue.

Successful practice scaling demands careful balance between growth ambition and quality maintenance, requiring strategic planning that protects client relationships while building sustainable competitive advantages. The most profitable consulting practices combine operational efficiency with strategic positioning that creates barriers to competition and premium pricing power.

From Solo Practice to Team Building

Team composition strategy requires understanding which functions can be delegated effectively while maintaining quality standards that protect professional reputation and client satisfaction. Not all consulting activities lend themselves to delegation, and inappropriate staffing decisions can destroy practices that took years to build.

Administrative support functions including scheduling, correspondence, and basic research can often be delegated to qualified support staff with appropriate training and supervision. However, analytical activities requiring clinical judgment and professional expertise typically require licensed professional involvement.

Staff qualification requirements for legal nurse consulting support positions include healthcare backgrounds, legal experience, or specialized training that enables effective contribution to consulting activities without compromising quality standards.

Medical records organization, preliminary research, and administrative coordination can be handled by staff with appropriate backgrounds and training. However, clinical analysis, opinion formation, and expert witness activities require licensed professional expertise that cannot be delegated safely.

Quality control systems for team-based practices require systematic supervision, review protocols, and accountability measures that ensure delegated work meets professional standards while protecting consultant reputation and client relationships.

Former emergency medicine nurse Dr. Patricia Thompson successfully scaled her practice from solo consulting to five-person team through systematic hiring and quality control development that maintained service excellence while increasing capacity.

Patricia's team development began with administrative assistant hiring to handle scheduling, correspondence, and basic research activities that consumed significant time without requiring clinical expertise. This delegation freed her to focus on analytical work that generated higher revenue.

Her second hire included a registered nurse with emergency department experience who could handle preliminary record review, timeline development, and basic research under Patricia's supervision. This addition doubled her case capacity without proportional cost increases.

The team expansion required systematic training programs, quality control procedures, and performance monitoring that ensured delegated work met Patricia's professional standards. Her investment in team development paid dividends through increased revenue and improved work-life balance.

Training and development programs for team members ensure consistent quality standards while building capabilities that support practice growth and service expansion.

Performance management systems provide accountability measures and improvement feedback that maintain quality standards while supporting professional development for team members.

Compensation structures for team-based practices must balance cost control with talent retention, often requiring creative approaches including profit sharing, performance bonuses, and professional development opportunities.

Subcontracting and Collaboration Models

Independent contractor relationships with other legal nurse consultants provide capacity expansion without employee overhead while maintaining flexibility for varying case loads and specialized expertise requirements.

Subcontracting arrangements require careful selection of qualified consultants whose work quality and professional standards align with your practice reputation. Poor subcontractor performance reflects directly on your professional credibility and client relationships.

Quality assurance protocols for subcontracted work must ensure consistent standards across all service delivery while maintaining client confidence in analysis quality and professional reliability.

Systematic review procedures, standardized deliverables, and performance monitoring help maintain quality standards while providing accountability measures for subcontracted consulting activities.

Specialization partnerships with consultants in complementary clinical areas create referral networks and collaboration opportunities that benefit all participants while providing clients access to specialized expertise.

Emergency medicine consultants might partner with surgical specialists, critical care experts, and toxicology consultants to handle complex cases requiring multiple clinical perspectives and specialized knowledge.

Former surgical nurse Dr. Michael Rodriguez built successful collaboration networks that enabled complex case handling while providing revenue sharing opportunities for participating consultants.

Michael's collaboration model included formal agreements with consultants in orthopedics, anesthesia, and critical care who could provide specialized analysis for complex surgical cases requiring multiple clinical perspectives.

The partnership agreements established clear roles, responsibility divisions, and compensation arrangements that protected all participants while ensuring quality service delivery for attorney clients.

His collaboration network enabled Michael to accept complex cases that exceeded his individual expertise while providing partners access to surgical litigation opportunities they couldn't handle independently.

Revenue sharing arrangements require careful structuring to ensure fair compensation while maintaining profitability and competitive pricing for attorney clients.

Client communication protocols for collaborative engagements ensure consistent messaging and professional presentation while maintaining clear accountability for deliverable quality and timeline compliance.

Conflict management procedures address disagreements about analysis approaches, case conclusions, and professional responsibilities that might arise during collaborative consulting engagements.

Multiple Revenue Streams Development

Service diversification beyond basic consulting creates multiple revenue sources while reducing dependence on traditional case analysis for practice sustainability and growth.

Expert witness services command premium pricing while requiring specialized skills and credentials that create competitive advantages and market differentiation opportunities.

Training and education services for attorney clients provide additional revenue while building relationships and demonstrating expertise through educational content delivery.

Legal nurse consultants can develop continuing education programs for law firms, educational seminars for bar associations, and specialized training courses that provide recurring revenue streams.

Product development opportunities include educational materials, analytical tools, and professional resources that generate passive income while building professional recognition and market presence.

Books, online courses, and professional templates provide revenue opportunities while establishing thought leadership and professional credibility that supports consulting practice development.

Former critical care nurse Dr. Jennifer Martinez diversified her practice revenue through systematic service expansion that reduced case analysis dependence while increasing total practice profitability.

Jennifer's diversification strategy included expert witness service development, educational program creation for attorney clients, and online course development for nurses entering legal consulting.

Her expert witness services commanded premium pricing while requiring specialized preparation and credentials that created competitive barriers and market differentiation.

The educational programs provided recurring revenue through continuing education presentations, while online courses generated passive income that continued growing without proportional time investment.

Passive income development through intellectual property creation provides ongoing revenue without direct time investment while building professional recognition and market presence.

Strategic partnerships with related service providers create referral opportunities and collaborative revenue streams that benefit all participants while expanding client service capabilities.

Technology monetization including software tools, analytical platforms, and professional resources can generate additional revenue while improving service delivery efficiency and client satisfaction.

Geographic Expansion Strategies

Market analysis for geographic expansion requires understanding regional litigation patterns, attorney practices, and competitive situations that affect expansion success and profitability potential.

Different geographic markets offer varying opportunities based on population density, litigation activity, and competitive intensity that affect revenue potential and market entry difficulty.

Virtual service delivery capabilities enable geographic expansion without physical presence requirements while maintaining cost efficiency and service quality for distant clients.

Remote consulting, virtual depositions, and electronic case management enable service delivery across wide geographic areas without travel expenses or physical office requirements.

Local partnership development with attorneys and consultants in target markets provides market entry assistance while building referral networks and professional relationships that support expansion success.

Regulatory compliance requirements vary by state and jurisdiction, requiring careful analysis of licensing, registration, and professional requirements that affect expansion feasibility and cost.

Former obstetric nurse Dr. Sandra Chen expanded her practice from regional to national scope through systematic geographic development that built market presence while maintaining service quality.

Sandra's expansion strategy included virtual service delivery capability development, partnership building with attorneys in target markets, and regulatory compliance research for multi-state practice.

Her virtual capabilities enabled case analysis and expert witness services for clients nationwide without travel requirements for most activities. Only deposition and trial testimony required physical presence in distant locations.

The expansion success required investment in technology infrastructure, professional marketing for distant markets, and relationship building with attorneys who couldn't evaluate her services through personal interaction.

Brand building for expanded markets requires consistent professional presentation and marketing messages that build recognition and credibility across wider geographic areas.

Quality maintenance across extended geographic markets requires systematic quality control and client communication that ensures consistent service delivery regardless of physical distance.

Cost management for geographic expansion includes technology investments, marketing expenses, and travel costs that affect profitability and pricing competitiveness in distant markets.

Technology Automation for Efficiency

Process automation opportunities include routine administrative tasks, document organization, and communication activities that can be streamlined through technology while maintaining quality standards.

Case management software, automated scheduling systems, and document processing tools can significantly reduce administrative overhead while improving service delivery efficiency and client satisfaction.

Artificial intelligence applications for preliminary analysis, pattern recognition, and quality checking can improve efficiency while maintaining analytical accuracy and professional standards.

AI tools can assist with initial document organization, timeline development, and preliminary analysis that supports detailed professional review without replacing clinical judgment and expertise.

Client communication automation including status updates, report delivery, and scheduling coordination can improve service responsiveness while reducing administrative overhead.

Quality control automation through systematic checking processes, verification protocols, and standardized deliverables helps maintain consistency while reducing manual oversight requirements.

Former cardiac care nurse Dr. Robert Kim implemented systematic automation that improved practice efficiency while maintaining quality standards and client satisfaction levels.

Robert's automation strategy included case management software implementation, automated time tracking systems, and standardized report templates that reduced administrative overhead while improving consistency.

His AI-assisted document organization enabled faster case setup and preliminary analysis, while automated client communication provided timely updates without manual coordination requirements.

The technology investments required initial capital and learning time but generated significant efficiency improvements that increased profitability while maintaining service quality standards.

ROI measurement for technology investments requires systematic tracking of efficiency gains, cost reductions, and revenue improvements that justify automation investments and guide future technology decisions.

Integration challenges between different software systems require careful planning and implementation that ensures smooth workflow and data consistency across technology platforms.

Security requirements for automated systems must maintain HIPAA compliance and client confidentiality while providing efficiency benefits and improved service delivery capabilities.

Exit Strategies and Practice Valuation

Practice valuation methods for legal nurse consulting businesses require understanding intangible asset values, client relationship worth, and revenue sustainability that affect sale price and buyer interest.

Legal nurse consulting practices depend heavily on personal relationships and professional reputation that may not transfer easily to new owners, affecting valuation and sale feasibility.

Succession planning options include employee buyouts, external sales, and gradual transition arrangements that provide exit opportunities while maintaining client relationships and practice value.

Client relationship transfer represents the biggest challenge in practice sales because attorney clients may prefer working with known consultants rather than accepting new service providers.

Asset identification for practice valuation includes client lists, intellectual property, systems and processes, and professional reputation that contribute to practice value and sale attractiveness.

Buyer qualification for legal nurse consulting practices requires understanding professional requirements, industry knowledge, and financial capabilities that ensure successful practice continuation.

Former emergency medicine nurse Dr. Lisa Park developed exit planning strategies that preserved practice value while providing multiple transition options for eventual practice sale or succession.

Lisa's exit planning included systematic documentation of processes and procedures, client relationship development that reduced personal dependency, and financial planning that supported retirement goals.

Her approach included training associates who could potentially buy the practice, developing referral relationships that could support practice transition, and building systems that reduced dependence on her personal involvement.

The systematic planning created multiple exit options while maintaining practice value and ensuring client service continuation regardless of transition timing or buyer characteristics.

Financial planning for practice exit requires understanding tax implications, valuation methods, and transition strategies that maximize financial return while ensuring smooth client relationship transfer.

Legal considerations for practice sales include contract transfers, liability assignments, and regulatory compliance that affect sale feasibility and buyer protection requirements.

Timeline development for exit strategies requires systematic planning that builds practice value while preparing for eventual transition without disrupting current operations or client relationships.

Growing Beyond Individual Limits

Practice scaling represents the natural evolution for successful legal nurse consultants who want to build lasting business value while reducing personal time investment in routine activities. The systematic approaches outlined here provide frameworks for growth that maintain quality standards while creating scalable business models.

Your success in scaling depends on careful balance between growth ambition and quality maintenance, requiring strategic thinking that protects what you've built while reaching for greater impact and financial return. Professional excellence and business acumen must work together to create sustainable competitive advantages.

Practice Scaling Strategies for Sustainable Growth

- Team building requires systematic hiring, training, and quality control that maintains service excellence while increasing capacity and reducing personal workload

- Subcontracting and collaboration models provide capacity expansion and specialization access while maintaining quality standards and competitive positioning

- Multiple revenue streams through service diversification reduce dependence on traditional consulting while creating passive income and competitive differentiation

- Geographic expansion through virtual delivery and local partnerships increases market access while maintaining cost efficiency and service quality

- Technology automation improves operational efficiency while maintaining quality standards and reducing administrative overhead for improved profitability

- Exit strategies and practice valuation planning preserve business value while creating transition options that protect client relationships and financial return

Chapter 15: Overcoming Common Challenges

Legal nurse consulting presents unique professional challenges that combine the emotional intensity of medical cases with the adversarial nature of litigation—creating stress patterns that traditional nursing careers never prepared you to handle. You'll face demanding attorneys, irregular income flows, aggressive cross-examination, and constant pressure to stay current with rapidly changing medical and legal standards.

These challenges can overwhelm even experienced consultants who lack systematic approaches to stress management, professional development, and business stability. The most successful legal nurse consultants develop resilience frameworks and problem-solving strategies that turn these challenges into competitive advantages rather than career-limiting obstacles.

Dealing with Difficult Cases and Demanding Attorneys

High-stress case management requires systematic approaches to emotional regulation and professional objectivity when analyzing tragic outcomes, preventable deaths, and cases involving children or particularly sympathetic plaintiffs.

Some cases involve emotional content that can trigger personal responses based on your clinical experiences or family situations. Pediatric deaths, preventable complications, and cases involving healthcare colleagues create particular challenges for maintaining analytical objectivity.

Professional boundary maintenance becomes essential when attorney clients pressure you for opinions beyond your expertise, demand unrealistic timelines, or request conclusions that exceed what evidence supports.

Attorneys facing trial deadlines or settlement pressures sometimes make unreasonable demands that could compromise your professional standards if not managed appropriately. Clear communication about professional limitations protects both your credibility and their case interests.

Difficult attorney personalities including aggressive communicators, demanding perfectionists, and those with unrealistic expectations require diplomatic management that maintains professional relationships while protecting your boundaries and work quality.

Some attorneys communicate in confrontational styles that work in courtroom settings but create stress in consultant relationships. Understanding these communication patterns helps you respond professionally without taking aggressive behavior personally.

Former surgical nurse Dr. Patricia Martinez faced a particularly challenging case involving a pediatric patient who died following routine appendectomy due to post-operative complications that her analysis suggested were preventable.

The case involved a seven-year-old child whose post-operative care included warning signs of developing complications that nursing staff failed to recognize or report appropriately. Patricia's analysis revealed multiple care standard violations that contributed to the child's death.

The emotional impact of analyzing preventable pediatric death challenged Patricia's professional objectivity, while the plaintiff attorney's aggressive timeline demands and pressure for definitive causation opinions exceeded reasonable professional expectations.

Patricia's coping strategy included peer consultation with experienced pediatric consultants, systematic documentation of her emotional responses and professional reasoning, and clear communication with the attorney about realistic timeline and opinion limitations.

Her professional boundary management included declining to provide opinions beyond nursing expertise, maintaining analytical objectivity despite emotional case content, and refusing to expedite analysis in ways that might compromise accuracy.

Stress management techniques for emotional case content include peer consultation, professional counseling resources, and systematic approaches to emotional regulation that prevent case content from affecting personal well-being.

Communication strategies for demanding attorneys include clear expectation setting, professional boundary explanation, and diplomatic resistance to unreasonable requests that maintain relationships while protecting professional standards.

Case selection criteria can help avoid consistently difficult situations by screening potential engagements for emotional content, timeline reasonableness, and attorney compatibility before accepting challenging cases.

Managing Irregular Income and Cash Flow

Income variability in legal nurse consulting creates financial planning challenges because case work arrives unpredictably and payment cycles often extend beyond normal business terms.

Legal cases develop irregularly based on litigation schedules, settlement negotiations, and court calendars that consultants cannot control. This unpredictability requires financial planning approaches that differ from regular employment income management.

Cash flow management requires systematic approaches to expense budgeting, income forecasting, and reserve fund maintenance that provide financial stability during slow periods or payment delays.

Emergency fund requirements for consulting practices often exceed those recommended for employees because income interruption can last several months during market downturns or seasonal variations.

Diversification strategies help stabilize income through multiple client relationships, different case types, and varied service offerings that reduce dependence on single income sources or client relationships.

Payment acceleration techniques including advance payments, progress billing, and invoice terms optimization can improve cash flow while maintaining client relationships and competitive positioning.

Former emergency medicine nurse Dr. Michael Rodriguez developed financial management systems that provided stability despite irregular consulting income and unpredictable payment cycles.

Michael's cash flow management included maintaining six months of living expenses in emergency reserves, diversifying client relationships across multiple law firms, and developing retainer arrangements that provided predictable monthly income.

His income stabilization strategy included offering different service levels with varying payment terms, developing recurring consulting relationships, and building expert witness capabilities that commanded premium pricing.

The systematic financial planning enabled Michael to weather slow periods without stress while maintaining investment in professional development and practice improvement during challenging financial cycles.

Budget planning for irregular income requires conservative projections, flexible expense management, and systematic saving during high-income periods to support low-income intervals.

Client payment management including clear terms, systematic invoicing, and professional collection procedures helps accelerate payment while maintaining positive client relationships.

Revenue forecasting based on historical patterns, current case pipeline, and market trends helps predict income variations and plan accordingly for business sustainability.

Staying Current with Medical and Legal Developments

Information overload challenges legal nurse consultants who must stay current with medical advances, legal developments, and professional standards across multiple specialty areas while maintaining productive consulting practice.

The volume of new information in healthcare and legal fields exceeds what any individual can process completely, requiring systematic approaches to priority setting and knowledge management.

Professional development planning requires strategic focus on information sources and educational activities that provide maximum value for consulting practice improvement and professional credibility building.

Continuing education investments must balance broad professional development with specialized knowledge that supports your specific consulting areas and competitive positioning.

Literature monitoring systems help track relevant developments through automated alerts, professional association updates, and systematic review of key journals and publications.

Technology tools including RSS feeds, journal alerts, and professional organization communications can help manage information flow while ensuring awareness of important developments affecting your practice areas.

Knowledge application strategies help translate new information into improved consulting services while avoiding the trap of constantly changing approaches based on every new development.

Former critical care nurse Dr. Jennifer Williams developed systematic approaches to professional currency that maintained current knowledge without overwhelming her consulting practice or creating analysis paralysis.

Jennifer's knowledge management system included monthly review of critical care journals, quarterly assessment of relevant legal developments, and annual evaluation of continuing education priorities based on practice needs.

Her systematic approach included automated journal alerts for specific topics, professional association newsletter review, and selective conference attendance based on strategic practice development goals.

The organized approach ensured currency with important developments while preventing information overload that could distract from productive consulting work and client service excellence.

Priority setting frameworks help identify which developments require immediate attention versus those that can be monitored without immediate action or knowledge integration.

Peer learning networks provide efficient ways to share information and learn from colleagues' experiences with new developments and their practical implications for consulting practice.

Technology tools for information management include databases, alert systems, and organization platforms that help track and apply new knowledge systematically.

Burnout Prevention in High-Stress Cases

Emotional exhaustion from exposure to medical tragedies, legal conflicts, and high-stakes litigation can accumulate over time without proper stress management and recovery strategies.

Legal nurse consulting combines the emotional demands of medical tragedy exposure with the adversarial stress of litigation, creating unique burnout risks that traditional nursing careers may not have prepared you to handle.

Work-life balance strategies help maintain perspective and emotional health while meeting the demanding requirements of complex consulting cases and aggressive litigation timelines.

Professional detachment techniques help maintain analytical objectivity while protecting emotional well-being when analyzing tragic cases or preventable outcomes.

Recovery period planning includes systematic breaks between intensive cases, stress management activities, and professional development that refreshes motivation and prevents accumulating emotional exhaustion.

Support system development including professional colleagues, personal relationships, and counseling resources provides outlets for stress management and emotional processing when needed.

Former obstetric nurse Dr. Sandra Chen implemented systematic burnout prevention strategies after recognizing early warning signs during particularly challenging periods involving multiple difficult cases.

Sandra's prevention approach included case load management that avoided simultaneous high-stress engagements, systematic vacation scheduling that provided recovery periods, and peer support relationships that offered professional consultation and emotional support.

Her stress management system included regular exercise, professional counseling when needed, and hobby development that provided mental and emotional balance outside consulting work.

The systematic approach prevented burnout while maintaining service excellence and professional satisfaction throughout challenging periods that could have overwhelmed consultants without proper support systems.

Warning sign recognition helps identify developing burnout before it affects professional performance or personal well-being significantly.

Stress reduction techniques including mindfulness practices, physical exercise, and relaxation activities provide systematic approaches to stress management and emotional regulation.

Professional counseling resources specifically trained in healthcare professional stress can provide specialized support for the unique challenges of legal nurse consulting.

Competitive Positioning and Differentiation

Market differentiation strategies help distinguish your services from numerous other legal nurse consultants competing for the same attorney clients and consulting opportunities.

Specialization advantages through clinical expertise, case type focus, or service offerings create competitive barriers while building recognition and referral opportunities.

Value proposition development clearly communicates unique benefits and competitive advantages that justify premium pricing or preferred consultant status with attorney clients.

Professional recognition through awards, publications, and speaking engagements builds credibility while creating competitive advantages that generic consultants cannot replicate easily.

Service innovation including new delivery methods, enhanced analysis approaches, or unique offerings provides competitive differentiation while improving client satisfaction and retention.

Former cardiac surgery nurse Dr. Robert Kim built competitive positioning through systematic specialization and professional recognition that created sustainable advantages over general consultants.

Robert's differentiation strategy focused on cardiac surgery and medical device expertise combined with published articles, conference presentations, and professional organization leadership that built recognition and credibility.

His specialized knowledge enabled premium pricing while creating referral patterns from attorneys who appreciated his unique qualifications and analytical depth.

The systematic positioning approach generated competitive advantages that protected against price competition while building sustainable client relationships and practice growth.

Brand building activities help create recognition and professional reputation that supports competitive positioning and premium pricing opportunities.

Client testimonial development provides third-party validation of service quality and competitive advantages that support marketing efforts and new client acquisition.

Continuous improvement processes ensure service excellence while adapting to changing market conditions and competitive pressures that affect practice sustainability.

Problem-Solving Frameworks for Complex Situations

Systematic analysis approaches help break down complex professional challenges into manageable components that can be addressed through logical problem-solving processes.

Decision-making frameworks provide structured approaches to difficult choices involving professional ethics, client relationships, and business decisions that affect practice success and professional reputation.

Resource identification helps locate appropriate assistance for challenges beyond individual expertise including legal counsel, professional consultation, and specialized support services.

Risk assessment procedures help evaluate potential consequences of different approaches while identifying mitigation strategies that protect professional and business interests.

Implementation planning ensures systematic execution of problem-solving decisions while monitoring outcomes and adjusting approaches based on results and changing circumstances.

Former emergency medicine nurse Dr. Lisa Park developed comprehensive problem-solving approaches that enabled effective handling of complex professional challenges throughout her consulting career.

Lisa's framework included systematic problem definition, stakeholder analysis, option evaluation, risk assessment, and implementation planning that provided consistent approaches to difficult situations.

Her resource network included professional colleagues, legal counsel, and business advisors who could provide specialized expertise for challenges beyond her individual knowledge and experience.

The systematic approach enabled confident decision-making during challenging situations while protecting her professional reputation and business interests throughout various complex circumstances.

Consultation resources including professional organizations, experienced colleagues, and specialized advisors provide support for complex problem-solving situations.

Documentation procedures help track problem-solving processes and decisions for future reference and professional protection during challenging situations.

Learning integration processes help extract lessons from difficult situations while building improved approaches for future challenge management and professional development.

Resilience Through Challenges

The challenges you'll face in legal nurse consulting are real and demanding, but they're also manageable through systematic approaches and professional development that builds resilience over time. Every successful consultant has faced similar challenges and developed coping strategies that turned obstacles into opportunities for growth and competitive advantage.

Your ability to handle these challenges professionally while maintaining service excellence and personal well-being determines your long-term success more than clinical expertise or initial market conditions. Build systematic approaches to challenge management that support both professional effectiveness and personal satisfaction.

Challenge Management Framework for Professional Resilience

- Difficult cases and demanding attorneys require professional boundary maintenance, stress management, and communication strategies that protect service quality while maintaining relationships

- Irregular income and cash flow challenges need systematic financial planning, diversification strategies, and payment management that provide stability despite unpredictable revenue patterns

- Staying current with medical and legal developments requires strategic information management, priority setting, and knowledge application that maintains currency without overwhelming practice demands

- Burnout prevention through work-life balance, stress management, and support system development protects emotional health while maintaining professional effectiveness

- Competitive positioning and differentiation create sustainable advantages through specialization, value proposition development, and professional recognition building

- Problem-solving frameworks provide systematic approaches to complex challenges while building resilience and professional growth through structured decision-making processes

Chapter 16: Navigating the Certification Maze

The legal nurse consulting certification process resembles a professional obstacle course designed by people who never had to actually practice in the field—requiring experience you can't get without certification and certification you can't obtain without experience. You'll discover that the alphabet soup of credentials (LNCC, CLNC, RN-LNC) creates more confusion than clarity for both new consultants and attorney clients trying to evaluate qualifications.

Most nurses approach certification decisions with the same systematic thinking they'd use for choosing breakfast cereal, yet these choices affect career trajectory, earning potential, and professional credibility for decades. Understanding the real-world implications of different certification paths helps you make strategic decisions that support long-term practice success rather than just checking professional boxes.

LNCC vs CLNC vs Other Certifications Compared

Legal Nurse Consultant Certified (LNCC) represents the gold standard certification from the American Association of Legal Nurse Consultants, requiring 2,000 hours of legal nurse consulting experience plus five years of nursing practice before you can even apply[65]. This creates the classic catch-22 that blocks entry for most aspiring consultants.

The LNCC examination covers legal concepts, case analysis, research methods, and professional practice standards through a rigorous testing process that many experienced consultants find challenging. Pass rates hover around 70%, and the certification requires renewal every five years with continuing education requirements.

However, the experience requirement means new consultants can't pursue LNCC certification immediately, forcing them to build practices without the credential that provides maximum professional recognition. This timing mismatch affects career planning and credibility building during early practice development.

Certified Legal Nurse Consultant (CLNC) from the National Alliance of Certified Legal Nurse Consultants offers more accessible entry requirements without the experience prerequisite that blocks LNCC eligibility. The certification focuses on practical skills through comprehensive training programs rather than experience-based qualification.

CLNC certification costs significantly less than university-based programs and can be completed in weeks rather than months or years. The program includes business development training, case analysis techniques, and marketing strategies that many consultants find practically useful for practice development.

However, CLNC recognition varies among attorneys and healthcare organizations, with some preferring the more rigorous LNCC credential despite its accessibility limitations. The marketing-heavy approach of some CLNC programs also creates skepticism among traditional nursing professionals.

RN-Legal Nurse Consultant (RN-LNC) certification from various organizations attempts to bridge the gap between nursing credentials and legal consulting qualifications through hybrid programs that recognize nursing experience while adding legal knowledge.

These programs typically require nursing licensure plus additional training in legal concepts, case analysis, and expert witness preparation. The requirements vary significantly between certifying organizations, creating confusion about qualification standards and professional recognition.

Former ICU nurse Dr. Patricia Martinez navigated the certification maze strategically, ultimately pursuing multiple credentials to maximize professional recognition and career flexibility throughout her consulting development.

Patricia initially chose CLNC certification because she couldn't meet LNCC experience requirements when starting her practice. The CLNC training provided practical business development skills and case analysis techniques that helped her establish client relationships and build experience.

After accumulating 2,000 hours of consulting experience over three years, Patricia pursued LNCC certification to gain maximum professional credibility and recognition. The rigorous examination process validated her knowledge while providing the gold standard credential that attorney clients respected most.

Her dual certification approach provided early practice entry through CLNC while building toward LNCC recognition that supported expert witness qualification and premium pricing as her practice matured.

Specialty certifications in clinical areas like critical care (CCRN), emergency medicine (CEN), or surgical nursing (CNOR) often provide more credibility with attorney clients than general legal nurse consulting credentials because they demonstrate specialized clinical expertise.

Academic credentials including bachelor's, master's, or doctoral degrees in nursing or related fields frequently carry more weight with attorney clients than certification programs, particularly for expert witness qualification and premium consulting opportunities.

Professional organization memberships in AALNC, specialty nursing associations, and state organizations provide continuing education and networking opportunities that support practice development regardless of certification choices.

Breaking the Experience-Certification Catch-22

Alternative experience pathways help build the consulting hours needed for LNCC certification through volunteer work, reduced-fee cases, and collaborative arrangements with experienced consultants who can provide mentorship and case opportunities.

Many experienced consultants need assistance with large cases and will provide subcontracting opportunities that count toward experience requirements while offering learning opportunities and professional development.

Pro bono work for legal aid organizations, public defender offices, and nonprofit organizations provides legitimate consulting experience while serving community needs and building professional relationships.

These organizations often need medical expertise for cases involving indigent clients but lack budgets for market-rate consulting fees. Pro bono work provides experience while demonstrating professional commitment to justice and community service.

Mentorship arrangements with experienced legal nurse consultants can provide guidance, case opportunities, and professional development that accelerates experience accumulation while building professional relationships.

Training case participation through continuing education programs sometimes provides simulated consulting experience that helps build skills and knowledge while creating networking opportunities with experienced consultants and attorney instructors.

Former emergency nurse Dr. Michael Rodriguez broke the experience barrier through strategic pro bono work and mentorship relationships that provided legitimate consulting experience while building professional networks.

Michael's strategy included volunteering with the local legal aid organization to review medical records for indigent clients, providing reduced-rate consulting for small firms that couldn't afford market rates, and collaborating with experienced consultants on complex cases.

His pro bono work with domestic violence cases provided experience with injury pattern analysis, medical record review, and expert witness preparation while serving an important community need.

The mentorship relationship with an established emergency medicine consultant provided access to overflow cases, professional guidance, and networking opportunities that accelerated his practice development while building toward LNCC qualification.

Documentation strategies for experience accumulation require systematic record-keeping that tracks consulting hours, case types, and activities that qualify toward certification requirements.

Case complexity building involves starting with simpler cases and gradually accepting more complex engagements that build skills while accumulating experience hours needed for certification eligibility.

Quality over quantity approaches focus on thorough case analysis and professional development rather than simply accumulating hours through minimal consulting activities.

Alternative Pathways to Credibility

Published writing in professional journals, legal publications, and online platforms builds credibility and professional recognition that often exceeds certification value for attorney clients seeking subject matter experts.

Articles about clinical topics affecting litigation, case studies demonstrating analytical approaches, and educational content addressing legal issues provide evidence of expertise while building professional visibility.

Speaking engagements at continuing education events, professional conferences, and bar association meetings demonstrate knowledge and communication skills while building relationships with potential clients and referral sources.

Teaching experience through universities, professional organizations, and continuing education providers builds credibility while demonstrating knowledge depth and communication abilities that attorneys value in consultants.

Professional awards and recognition from nursing organizations, legal associations, and community groups provide third-party validation of expertise and professional excellence.

Board certification in nursing specialties relevant to your consulting practice often carries more weight with attorney clients than general legal nurse consulting credentials because it demonstrates clinical expertise depth.

Former surgical nurse Dr. Jennifer Williams built credibility through systematic professional development that created recognition and opportunities without relying solely on certification credentials.

Jennifer's credibility building included publishing articles about surgical complications in legal nursing journals, presenting educational programs about operating room standards at bar association meetings, and teaching surgical nursing courses at the local university.

Her professional recognition included selection as Expert Nurse of the Year from the state nursing organization, appointment to the hospital medical staff committee on surgical quality, and invitation to serve on professional organization boards.

The systematic credibility building created professional recognition that exceeded certification value while establishing her as a recognized expert in surgical nursing and legal consulting.

Portfolio development showcasing education, experience, publications, and professional achievements provides concrete evidence of qualifications that supplements or replaces certification credentials.

Professional networking through multiple organizations and communities builds relationships and recognition that often matter more than certification status for practice development and client acquisition.

Continuing education documentation demonstrates ongoing professional development and knowledge currency that attorney clients value for case analysis and expert witness services.

Continuing Education Requirements and Opportunities

LNCC maintenance requires 30 contact hours of continuing education every five years, with specific requirements for legal, nursing, and general professional development topics that maintain knowledge currency across multiple disciplines.

The education must include legal updates, clinical practice developments, and professional skills training that support effective consulting practice and expert witness qualification.

CLNC renewal typically involves shorter continuing education requirements focused on case analysis skills, business development, and professional practice updates rather than extensive academic requirements.

Nursing license maintenance requires continuing education that varies by state but typically includes clinical updates, professional development, and specialty training that maintains competence for clinical practice background.

Professional development planning helps identify educational priorities based on practice needs, client feedback, and industry trends that affect consulting effectiveness and competitive positioning.

Educational resource evaluation includes assessing continuing education providers, program quality, and cost-effectiveness for professional development investment and certification maintenance.

Former critical care nurse Dr. Sandra Chen developed systematic continuing education strategies that exceeded certification requirements while building specialized knowledge that supported practice growth and expert witness development.

Sandra's education planning included annual assessment of learning needs based on practice feedback, client requirements, and industry developments affecting critical care litigation.

Her educational portfolio included university courses in legal studies, specialized training in medical device technology, and advanced certification in critical care nursing that built expertise depth.

The systematic approach ensured knowledge currency while building credentials that supported expert witness qualification and premium pricing for specialized consulting services.

Cost-benefit analysis for continuing education investments helps prioritize spending on activities that provide maximum professional development return while meeting certification requirements efficiently.

Time management for continuing education requires balancing practice demands with learning requirements through strategic scheduling and efficient educational resource utilization.

Knowledge application strategies help translate continuing education into improved consulting services while building competitive advantages and client satisfaction.

Professional Portfolio Development

Credential documentation requires systematic organization of education, experience, certifications, and professional achievements in formats that support client evaluation and expert witness qualification.

Professional portfolios should include detailed curriculum vitae, case experience summaries, publication lists, and professional references that demonstrate qualifications and credibility.

Case experience presentation showcases consulting engagements and expert witness testimony through case studies that demonstrate analytical capabilities without violating confidentiality requirements.

Publication compilation includes articles, research papers, and professional writing that demonstrates expertise while building professional recognition and thought leadership.

Professional reference development involves building relationships with attorney clients, nursing colleagues, and professional contacts who can provide credible testimonials about service quality and professional competence.

Visual presentation of portfolio materials through professional formatting, organization, and presentation helps create positive impressions with attorney clients evaluating consultant qualifications.

Former obstetric nurse Dr. Robert Kim developed professional portfolios that effectively communicated his qualifications while supporting business development and expert witness marketing efforts.

Robert's portfolio included detailed sections on education and training, clinical experience with obstetric complications, legal consulting case summaries, and expert witness testimony record.

His case studies showcased analytical approaches and opinion development without revealing confidential information, demonstrating expertise while protecting client confidentiality and professional ethics.

The professional presentation included high-quality formatting, clear organization, and compelling content that helped attorney clients understand his qualifications and service capabilities.

Digital portfolio development through professional websites and online platforms provides accessible qualification information while supporting marketing efforts and client evaluation processes.

Portfolio maintenance requires regular updates with new experience, education, and achievements that keep qualification information current and comprehensive.

Customization strategies help tailor portfolio presentation to specific client needs, case types, and expert witness opportunities that maximize qualification impact.

Networking and Professional Relationships

Strategic relationship building requires systematic approaches to professional networking that create mutual value while building referral opportunities and professional support systems.

Effective networking focuses on relationship development rather than immediate business generation, building trust and familiarity that supports long-term practice growth and professional recognition.

Professional organization participation through AALNC, specialty nursing associations, and legal organizations provides networking opportunities while building professional visibility and credibility.

Mentorship relationships work both ways—serving as mentor to newer consultants while continuing to learn from experienced professionals who can provide guidance and opportunities.

Cross-referral networks with consultants in different specialties create mutual support systems that benefit all participants while providing clients access to specialized expertise.

Attorney relationship cultivation through consistent professional service, value-added communication, and relationship maintenance creates client loyalty and referral generation.

Former pediatric nurse Dr. Lisa Park built professional networks that supported practice growth while providing professional development and referral opportunities throughout her consulting career.

Lisa's networking strategy included active participation in AALNC local chapters, leadership roles in pediatric nursing organizations, and attendance at legal conferences focused on child-related litigation.

Her mentorship approach included guidance for new legal nurse consultants while continuing professional development through relationships with experienced experts in pediatric medicine and legal consulting.

The cross-referral relationships with consultants in adolescent psychiatry, child development, and educational psychology created collaboration opportunities while providing specialized expertise for complex cases.

Relationship maintenance requires systematic follow-up, value-added communication, and professional support that builds lasting connections beyond immediate business needs.

Professional reputation management involves consistent service excellence, ethical practice, and professional development that builds positive recognition within professional communities.

Networking efficiency strategies help maximize relationship building impact while managing time investment and maintaining authentic professional connections.

The Path Forward

Certification represents just one component of professional credibility in legal nurse consulting—often less important than experience, specialized knowledge, and professional relationships that demonstrate competence and trustworthiness. The most successful consultants focus on building genuine expertise and professional recognition rather than simply collecting credentials.

Your certification decisions should align with long-term career goals while recognizing that professional success depends more on service quality and relationship building than credential accumulation. Build systematic approaches to professional development that support both immediate practice needs and future growth opportunities.

Certification Strategy Framework for Professional Development

- LNCC provides maximum professional recognition but requires 2,000 hours of experience that creates entry barriers for new consultants seeking immediate credibility

- CLNC offers accessible entry without experience requirements but may lack recognition among some attorney clients and professional organizations

- Alternative credibility pathways through publication, speaking, teaching, and professional recognition often provide more value than certification credentials

- Continuing education requirements for certification maintenance should align with practice development needs and professional growth objectives

- Professional portfolio development requires systematic documentation of qualifications, experience, and achievements that support client evaluation and expert witness marketing

- Networking and professional relationships provide more practice development value than certification status through referral generation and professional support systems

Chapter 17: Future-Proofing Your LNC Career

The healthcare and legal industries stand on the precipice of technological revolution that will fundamentally alter how legal nurse consulting operates—yet most consultants approach career planning as if nothing will change in the next decade. Artificial intelligence, regulatory transformation, and evolving healthcare delivery models create both unprecedented opportunities and existential threats that require strategic adaptation rather than passive response.

You can either position yourself at the forefront of these changes and capture the benefits of early adoption, or you can resist until market forces make adaptation necessary for survival. The consultants who thrive in the coming decades will be those who understand these trends and build capabilities that complement rather than compete with technological advancement.

Industry Trends and Adaptation Strategies

Healthcare digitization acceleration continues transforming medical practice through electronic health records, telemedicine platforms, and AI-assisted diagnostics that create new liability patterns requiring specialized legal expertise[66]. These technological implementations generate novel malpractice scenarios that traditional experts cannot analyze effectively.

The shift toward value-based care models rather than fee-for-service creates different incentive structures and quality metrics that affect malpractice standards and expert witness requirements. Legal nurse consultants must understand these evolving payment models and their impact on care delivery decisions.

Remote healthcare delivery expansion beyond pandemic emergency measures creates permanent changes in care standards, technology dependencies, and liability frameworks that require specialized knowledge for effective case analysis[67]. Telehealth malpractice represents a rapidly growing specialty area with minimal expert competition.

Regulatory compliance complexity increases as healthcare systems face mounting requirements for quality reporting, patient safety monitoring, and outcome transparency that create new categories of institutional liability and expert witness needs.

The aging population demographic shift creates increased demand for geriatric care expertise, elder abuse investigation, and nursing home liability analysis that represent growth opportunities for consultants with appropriate clinical backgrounds.

Former cardiac surgery nurse Dr. Patricia Thompson adapted her practice proactively by developing expertise in minimally invasive surgical techniques and robotic surgery complications that became increasingly common in cardiac litigation as technology adoption accelerated.

Patricia's adaptation strategy included completing additional training in robotic surgical systems, attending manufacturer training programs, and developing relationships with engineers who could explain technical failures during litigation.

Her early expertise in robotic surgery complications positioned her as one of few consultants who could analyze cases involving new surgical technologies, creating premium pricing opportunities and reduced competition in this specialized area.

The strategic positioning required ongoing education investment and technology learning that exceeded traditional nursing requirements, but the competitive advantages justified the additional effort and expense.

Workforce shortage impacts in healthcare create staffing-related liability issues, scope-of-practice expansion questions, and quality concerns that generate litigation requiring specialized nursing expertise about staffing standards and care delivery models.

Healthcare consolidation trends toward larger health systems create different organizational structures, policy frameworks, and liability patterns that require understanding of corporate healthcare management and quality systems.

Patient safety movement expansion creates more sophisticated quality monitoring, incident reporting, and risk management systems that affect litigation evidence and expert analysis requirements.

Technology Integration and AI Collaboration

Artificial intelligence adoption in healthcare creates diagnostic assistance, treatment recommendations, and clinical decision support that can fail in ways requiring expert analysis about appropriate technology use and human oversight requirements[68].

AI diagnostic errors represent emerging liability categories when algorithmic systems fail to identify diseases, recommend inappropriate treatments, or provide biased results that harm patients. Legal nurse consultants who understand both clinical care and AI limitations become essential for these cases.

Electronic health record complexity continues increasing as systems integrate more data sources, decision support tools, and automation features that can malfunction or create user errors requiring specialized analysis[69].

EHR-related errors include medication dosing mistakes from automated calculations, missed diagnoses from alert fatigue, and communication failures from system design problems that require technical understanding for effective analysis.

Data security and privacy concerns create new liability categories when healthcare organizations suffer breaches, ransomware attacks, or system failures that affect patient care quality and safety[70].

Cybersecurity incidents that disrupt clinical operations can cause medication errors, delayed treatments, and communication breakdowns requiring analysis of both technology failures and clinical response adequacy.

Wearable technology integration into healthcare monitoring creates liability questions when devices fail, provide inaccurate data, or create false alarms that affect treatment decisions and patient outcomes.

Former emergency medicine nurse Dr. Michael Rodriguez positioned his practice for AI-era opportunities by developing expertise in emergency department technology systems and their failure modes during clinical decision-making processes.

Michael's technology education included training in emergency department information systems, clinical decision support tools, and AI-assisted diagnostic systems that were becoming standard in emergency medicine practice.

His expertise in technology-assisted emergency care enabled analysis of cases involving system failures, user errors, and inappropriate reliance on automated recommendations that contributed to patient harm.

The specialized knowledge positioned Michael as one of few consultants who could analyze complex cases involving multiple technology systems and their interactions during emergency care delivery.

Blockchain applications in healthcare for secure data sharing and patient record management create new technical infrastructure that can fail in ways requiring expert analysis about appropriate implementation and monitoring.

Predictive analytics use in healthcare for risk assessment and treatment planning creates liability questions when algorithms recommend inappropriate interventions or fail to identify high-risk patients appropriately.

Robotic technology expansion beyond surgery into medication management, patient monitoring, and care delivery creates new failure modes requiring analysis of human-machine interaction and oversight requirements.

Regulatory Changes and Compliance Requirements

Quality reporting mandates continue expanding through Medicare and Medicaid requirements, accreditation standards, and state regulations that create new compliance obligations and liability exposure for healthcare organizations.

These reporting requirements generate extensive documentation that becomes evidence in litigation while creating new standards for quality measurement and institutional accountability.

Patient safety regulations evolve through Joint Commission updates, Centers for Medicare & Medicaid Services requirements, and state oversight that affect care standards and institutional liability exposure.

Scope of practice expansions for nurses, physician assistants, and other healthcare professionals create liability questions about appropriate supervision, training requirements, and competency validation that require expert analysis.

Advanced practice nurses assuming responsibilities previously limited to physicians face different liability standards and practice requirements that affect malpractice analysis and expert witness qualifications.

Telehealth regulatory frameworks continue developing as states establish licensing requirements, standard-of-care guidelines, and liability frameworks for remote healthcare delivery[71].

Interstate practice licensing compacts change how healthcare professionals can practice across state lines, affecting liability jurisdiction and applicable care standards for telehealth services.

Former critical care nurse Dr. Jennifer Williams adapted her practice to regulatory changes by developing expertise in ICU staffing regulations and quality reporting requirements that became central to critical care malpractice cases.

Jennifer's regulatory expertise included understanding nurse-to-patient ratio requirements, monitoring standards for different acuity levels, and quality indicators used for ICU performance measurement.

Her knowledge of regulatory frameworks enabled analysis of institutional liability related to staffing violations, quality reporting failures, and compliance deficiencies that contributed to patient harm.

The specialized regulatory knowledge created competitive advantages in cases involving institutional policy violations and systematic care failures rather than individual provider negligence.

Privacy law evolution through HIPAA updates, state privacy statutes, and technology-specific regulations affects healthcare data handling and creates new liability categories for privacy violations.

Professional licensing changes including continuing education requirements, competency validation, and scope limitations affect individual practitioner liability and expert witness qualification standards.

Healthcare fraud prevention through increased oversight, whistleblower protections, and compliance monitoring creates new legal categories requiring medical expertise for case analysis.

Market Expansion Opportunities

International healthcare litigation creates opportunities for consultants with expertise in global health systems, medical tourism complications, and cross-border care quality standards.

Medical tourism cases involving complications from overseas procedures require understanding of different healthcare systems, quality standards, and legal frameworks that affect liability analysis.

Healthcare technology exports create liability exposure when American medical devices, pharmaceuticals, or systems cause harm in international markets requiring expert analysis about design standards and user training.

Consulting firm partnerships with major accounting firms, management consultancies, and technology companies create opportunities for healthcare expertise in business contexts beyond traditional litigation.

Government consulting opportunities through Medicare fraud investigation, regulatory compliance assessment, and policy development require healthcare expertise in administrative and regulatory contexts.

Corporate healthcare clients including health systems, insurance companies, and technology companies need healthcare expertise for risk management, policy development, and strategic planning beyond litigation support.

Former surgical nurse Dr. Sandra Chen expanded her practice internationally by developing expertise in medical device regulation and surgical training standards that applied to global markets and cross-border litigation.

Sandra's international expansion included consulting on medical device failures affecting multiple countries, surgical training adequacy for device adoption, and regulatory compliance across different healthcare systems.

Her global expertise enabled premium consulting fees while creating competitive barriers through specialized knowledge that few consultants possessed about international healthcare systems and regulation.

The expansion required significant investment in regulatory education and relationship building but created sustainable competitive advantages and revenue diversification.

Healthcare policy consulting for government agencies, professional organizations, and advocacy groups provides opportunities to influence systemic changes while building professional recognition and expertise.

Health technology assessment for new medical devices, pharmaceuticals, and treatment protocols requires clinical expertise combined with economic analysis and policy understanding.

Academic partnerships with universities and research institutions create opportunities for healthcare expertise in research contexts, grant applications, and policy development projects.

Personal Branding and Thought Leadership

Content creation through articles, blogs, and professional publications builds recognition while demonstrating expertise that attracts consulting opportunities and speaking engagements.

Thought leadership requires consistent content production that addresses emerging trends, controversial issues, and practical solutions that resonate with target audiences.

Social media presence through LinkedIn, Twitter, and professional platforms creates visibility while building professional networks and demonstrating expertise to potential clients and referral sources.

Professional social media requires strategic content planning, consistent engagement, and reputation management that builds credibility while avoiding professional pitfalls.

Speaking circuit development through conferences, webinars, and professional events creates recognition while building expertise demonstration and professional networking opportunities.

Media relationships with healthcare reporters, legal journalists, and industry publications create opportunities for expert commentary that builds recognition and credibility.

Professional awards and recognition through nominations, applications, and peer recognition create third-party validation of expertise and professional excellence.

Former obstetric nurse Dr. Robert Kim built thought leadership through systematic content creation and speaking engagements that established him as recognized expert in maternal-fetal medicine litigation.

Robert's thought leadership strategy included monthly articles about obstetric complications for legal publications, quarterly speaking engagements at medical and legal conferences, and regular social media content addressing current issues in maternal care.

His media relationships included serving as expert source for healthcare reporters covering maternal mortality, pregnancy complications, and obstetric liability issues.

The systematic approach to thought leadership created professional recognition that generated consulting opportunities, speaking fees, and expert witness engagements that exceeded traditional practice revenue.

Intellectual property development through books, courses, and professional resources creates passive income while building professional recognition and expertise demonstration.

Professional association leadership through board service, committee participation, and volunteer activities creates recognition while building professional networks and industry influence.

Mentorship and teaching activities build professional legacy while creating recognition and relationship networks that support long-term career development.

Legacy Building and Industry Contribution

Professional mentorship of new legal nurse consultants ensures knowledge transfer while building professional relationships and industry reputation for guidance and support.

Effective mentorship requires systematic approaches to knowledge sharing, relationship development, and professional guidance that benefit both mentors and mentees.

Industry standard development through professional organizations, regulatory input, and best practice creation contributes to profession advancement while building personal recognition and influence.

Education program development for universities, professional organizations, and continuing education providers creates lasting impact while building expertise demonstration and professional legacy.

Research contribution through studies, data analysis, and publication creates knowledge advancement while building professional recognition and academic credibility.

Professional organization leadership provides opportunities to influence industry direction while building recognition and creating lasting impact on profession development.

Former pediatric nurse Dr. Lisa Park built professional legacy through systematic mentorship programs and industry contribution that influenced profession development while creating lasting recognition.

Lisa's legacy building included formal mentorship programs for new pediatric consultants, leadership roles in professional organizations, and development of educational resources for pediatric legal nurse consulting.

Her industry contributions included research on pediatric malpractice trends, development of best practice guidelines for child abuse investigation, and creation of continuing education programs for healthcare and legal professionals.

The systematic approach to legacy building created lasting impact while building professional recognition that exceeded individual practice success through industry influence and knowledge contribution.

Knowledge documentation through books, articles, and professional resources ensures expertise preservation while creating passive income and professional recognition.

Community service through pro bono work, volunteer activities, and public health contribution creates social impact while building professional reputation and personal satisfaction.

Innovation development through new methodologies, analytical approaches, and service delivery models contributes to profession advancement while creating competitive advantages and recognition.

Your Professional Horizon

The future of legal nurse consulting belongs to practitioners who combine clinical expertise with technological sophistication, strategic thinking, and adaptive capabilities that respond to changing market conditions. Success requires continuous learning, strategic positioning, and professional development that builds lasting competitive advantages.

Your career longevity depends on understanding industry trends while building capabilities that complement technological advancement rather than competing with automation. Position yourself as the human expert who provides context, judgment, and wisdom that technology cannot replicate.

Future-Proofing Strategies for Sustainable Success

- Industry trend awareness and adaptation strategies position consultants to capture benefits of healthcare digitization, regulatory changes, and demographic shifts

- Technology integration and AI collaboration create opportunities for consultants who understand both clinical care and technological limitations affecting patient safety

- Regulatory change monitoring and compliance expertise provide competitive advantages as healthcare faces increasing oversight and accountability requirements

- Market expansion opportunities through international consulting, government work, and corporate partnerships diversify revenue while building specialized expertise

- Personal branding and thought leadership create professional recognition and competitive advantages through content creation and expert positioning

- Legacy building through mentorship, industry contribution, and knowledge development creates lasting impact while building professional recognition and influence

Appendix A: Essential Templates and Checklists

Professional templates and systematic checklists separate successful legal nurse consultants from those who struggle with inconsistent quality and missed opportunities. You need proven frameworks that ensure thorough analysis, professional presentation, and systematic approaches to every aspect of consulting practice—from initial record review through expert witness preparation.

These tools represent the accumulated wisdom of successful practitioners who learned through trial and error what works in real-world consulting situations. Rather than reinventing approaches for every case, you can build on proven frameworks while adapting them to specific client needs and case requirements.

Medical Record Review Checklist

Pre-Review Organization establishes systematic approaches that prevent oversight and ensure thorough case analysis from the beginning. This foundational phase determines the quality and efficiency of your entire analytical process.

1. **Record Inventory Verification**

   - Count total pages received and verify completeness

   - Identify all healthcare providers and institutions involved

   - Check for missing time periods or care episodes

   - Document any illegible or damaged pages requiring clarification

- o Create master list of all record sources with page counts

2. **Chronological Organization**

   - o Sort all records by date and time of service
   - o Separate records by provider type (hospital, physician, laboratory, imaging)
   - o Create preliminary timeline of significant events
   - o Identify overlapping care periods requiring careful analysis
   - o Flag any chronological inconsistencies for investigation

3. **Key Personnel Identification**

   - o List all physicians involved in patient care
   - o Identify nursing staff by name and shift
   - o Note consultants and specialists who provided care
   - o Document administrative personnel involved in care decisions
   - o Create contact information database for potential depositions

Systematic Review Process ensures consistent analytical quality while preventing overlooked details that could affect case outcomes or professional credibility.

1. **Initial Assessment Phase**

   - o Review chief complaint and presenting symptoms
   - o Identify primary diagnoses and treatment plans
   - o Note any chronic conditions affecting care decisions

- o   Document medication history and allergies
- o   Assess patient compliance and social factors

2. **Care Standard Analysis**

   - o   Compare actual care against applicable protocols
   - o   Identify policy violations or guideline deviations
   - o   Research current literature supporting care standards
   - o   Document any experimental or unusual treatments
   - o   Note communication breakdowns between providers

3. **Outcome Analysis**

   - o   Trace progression from admission to discharge
   - o   Identify complications and their timing
   - o   Analyze response to treatments and interventions
   - o   Document any unexpected outcomes or deterioration
   - o   Assess whether outcomes were preventable

Former ICU nurse Dr. Patricia Martinez used this systematic checklist during analysis of a post-operative sepsis case that involved care across multiple units over two weeks. Her methodical approach revealed critical gaps in antibiotic therapy monitoring that other consultants had missed.

Patricia's checklist-driven review identified a 12-hour period where no nursing assessments were documented despite patient complaints of increasing pain and fever. The systematic approach helped her trace the infection progression and identify specific care failures that contributed to sepsis development.

Her detailed documentation of the review process provided credibility during deposition when opposing counsel questioned her analytical methods. The systematic approach demonstrated thorough preparation while protecting against challenges about overlooked evidence.

Quality Assurance Verification provides final accuracy checks that protect professional credibility and ensure deliverable quality before client submission.

1. **Factual Accuracy Review**
   - Verify all dates, times, and medical facts
   - Cross-check medication names and dosages
   - Confirm laboratory values and normal ranges
   - Validate timeline accuracy across multiple sources
   - Review medical terminology and spelling

2. **Analysis Completeness Check**
   - Ensure all relevant issues are addressed
   - Verify care standard research is current
   - Confirm causation analysis is supported
   - Review opinion formation reasoning
   - Check for any overlooked complications

3. **Professional Presentation Standards**
   - Review formatting and organization consistency
   - Check grammar and professional language use
   - Verify client confidentiality protection

- o Ensure appropriate medical terminology explanations
- o Confirm report meets contracted deliverable requirements

Case Analysis Templates

Executive Summary Template provides attorneys with essential case information in formats that support quick decision-making and strategy development. This section should answer key liability questions within the first two paragraphs.

Case Overview Format:

- Patient demographics and relevant medical history
- Key healthcare providers and institutions involved
- Timeline of significant events and complications
- Primary liability issues and care standard violations
- Causation analysis and damage assessment summary
- Case strengths and potential challenges identification

Detailed Analysis Structure organizes complex medical information in logical sequences that build legal arguments while maintaining clinical accuracy and professional credibility.

1. **Background and Medical History Section**
   - o Present relevant past medical history affecting current care
   - o Summarize social factors influencing treatment decisions

- o Document medication history and known allergies

- o Identify baseline functional status and quality of life

- o Note any previous similar episodes or complications

2. **Care Standard Analysis Section**

   - o Define applicable care standards for each time period

   - o Compare actual care provided against established protocols

   - o Identify specific policy violations or guideline deviations

   - o Document literature supporting care standard positions

   - o Address any alternative approaches or emergency modifications

3. **Causation Analysis Section**

   - o Establish timeline connecting care failures to patient harm

   - o Address alternative explanations for adverse outcomes

   - o Analyze contribution percentages for multiple factors

   - o Document preventability assessment for complications

   - o Review proximate cause relationships between acts and outcomes

Former emergency medicine nurse Dr. Michael Rodriguez developed template modifications for emergency department cases that addressed the unique challenges of crisis care analysis and protocol variations during emergency situations.

Michael's emergency-specific template included sections for triage decision analysis, resource availability assessment, and emergency protocol compliance that recognized the different care standards applicable during crisis situations.

His template addressed the challenge of incomplete documentation common in emergency settings while maintaining analytical rigor and professional standards for opinion formation and causation analysis.

The specialized template helped him complete emergency medicine cases more efficiently while ensuring consistent quality and professional presentation across different case types and complexity levels.

Opinion Formation Framework provides systematic approaches to professional opinion development that maintain objectivity while building credible conclusions supported by evidence and professional standards.

1. **Evidence Integration Process**
   - Synthesize findings from record review and research
   - Weight different evidence sources appropriately
   - Address contradictory information or conflicting evidence
   - Document reasoning process for opinion formation
   - Identify limitations or uncertainties in available evidence

2. **Professional Opinion Structure**

- State opinions clearly with appropriate qualification language
- Provide supporting reasoning for each conclusion
- Address alternative interpretations or explanations
- Acknowledge limitations of available evidence
- Maintain objectivity while providing definitive guidance

Contract Templates

Service Agreement Framework establishes clear business relationships while protecting consultant interests and ensuring client understanding of service scope and limitations.

Essential Contract Elements:

- Detailed scope of work descriptions and deliverable specifications
- Payment terms including rates, billing schedules, and late payment penalties
- Timeline requirements with milestone dates and deadline management
- Confidentiality obligations and work product protection clauses
- Liability limitations and professional responsibility boundaries
- Dispute resolution procedures and governing law provisions

Independent Contractor Language protects both parties from unintended employment relationships while clarifying professional service arrangements and tax obligations.

Key Protection Clauses:

- Clear independent contractor status definition

- Intellectual property ownership and usage rights

- Client materials return and destruction requirements

- Professional liability insurance acknowledgment

- Termination procedures and final payment arrangements

- Amendment requirements and contract modification procedures

Specialized Agreement Types address different consulting arrangements including expert witness services, training programs, and ongoing consultation relationships.

1. **Expert Witness Agreement Additions**

   o Qualification standards and credibility requirements

   o Testimony preparation time and compensation structure

   o Travel arrangements and expense reimbursement policies

   o Cancellation fees and short-notice change procedures

   o Deposition and trial testimony fee structures

2. **Retainer Agreement Modifications**

   o Monthly retainer amounts and service inclusions

   o Additional service billing procedures and rate structures

   o Availability requirements and response time expectations

   o Unused retainer credit and rollover policies

    o   Relationship termination and final billing procedures

Former surgical nurse Dr. Jennifer Williams learned contract importance through early career payment disputes that led to systematic contract development and professional legal review for all service agreements.

Jennifer's contract evolution included payment protection clauses after experiencing collection difficulties with slow-paying attorney clients, scope limitation language following expansion requests without additional compensation, and liability protection after facing threats of malpractice claims.

Her systematic contract approach prevented recurring problems while maintaining positive client relationships through clear expectation setting and professional boundary management.

Marketing Materials Examples

Professional Biography Template communicates qualifications and expertise in formats that attorney clients find useful for evaluation and decision-making processes.

Biography Structure:

- Opening statement highlighting unique qualifications and experience

- Education credentials with relevant specializations and honors

- Clinical experience summary emphasizing litigation-relevant background

- Legal consulting experience and case type specializations

- Professional affiliations and continuing education activities

- Publications, presentations, and professional recognition achievements

Service Description Framework explains consulting capabilities in clear language that helps attorney clients understand value propositions and engagement benefits.

Service Categories:

- Medical record analysis and case evaluation services
- Expert witness consultation and testimony preparation
- Healthcare policy analysis and regulatory compliance review
- Staff training and educational program development
- Quality assurance consulting and risk management analysis
- Specialized clinical expertise in particular medical areas

Client Testimonial Guidelines provide frameworks for collecting and presenting client feedback that builds credibility while maintaining professional confidentiality and ethical boundaries.

Testimonial Development Process:

- Request feedback systematically after successful case completion
- Provide template formats that highlight specific service benefits
- Ensure confidentiality protection and client consent for usage
- Focus on professional service quality rather than case outcomes
- Include attorney credentials and firm information when appropriate
- Update testimonials regularly to maintain current relevance

Expert Witness Preparation Guides

Qualification Preparation Checklist ensures systematic readiness for qualification challenges and credibility assessment during deposition and trial testimony.

1. **Credential Verification Process**

   - Update curriculum vitae with recent experience and education

   - Organize supporting documentation for all claimed qualifications

   - Prepare explanations for any gaps or career changes

   - Research current literature supporting analytical approaches

   - Review previous testimony transcripts for consistency verification

2. **Case-Specific Preparation Requirements**

   - Master all case facts and timeline details

   - Research applicable care standards and guideline updates

   - Prepare visual aids and demonstrative materials

   - Practice technical explanations for lay audiences

   - Anticipate cross-examination challenges and prepare responses

Testimony Performance Framework provides systematic approaches to effective communication during deposition and trial proceedings.

Communication Guidelines:

- Listen carefully to questions and answer only what is asked

- Use clear, simple language appropriate for jury understanding

- Maintain professional composure under aggressive questioning

- Acknowledge limitations and uncertainties appropriately

- Provide concrete examples to illustrate abstract concepts

- Project confidence while avoiding arrogance or defensiveness

Cross-Examination Survival Strategies prepare witnesses for aggressive questioning designed to discredit qualifications and challenge opinion accuracy.

Defense Techniques:

- Prepare responses to common impeachment attempts

- Practice staying calm under pressure and personal attacks

- Develop strategies for handling document confrontations

- Learn to redirect hostile questions toward favorable evidence

- Master techniques for acknowledging errors without losing credibility

- Prepare recovery methods for unexpected challenges or surprises

Former critical care nurse Dr. Sandra Chen developed expert witness preparation systems that helped her survive particularly aggressive cross-examination while maintaining credibility and opinion strength during high-stakes litigation.

Sandra's preparation included mock cross-examination sessions with attorneys, detailed research of opposing expert qualifications and previous testimony, and systematic practice with challenging questions about her methodology and conclusions.

Her systematic approach helped her maintain composure during four-hour cross-examination in a $5 million medical device case where opposing counsel attacked every aspect of her qualifications and analytical approach.

The thorough preparation enabled confident responses that actually strengthened her credibility while demonstrating the thoroughness of her analysis and the reliability of her professional opinions.

Building Your Success Foundation

These templates and checklists represent the operational foundation for professional legal nurse consulting practice. They provide systematic approaches that ensure quality while improving efficiency and protecting against the common mistakes that damage consultant credibility and client relationships.

Your success depends on developing consistent approaches that maintain quality standards while adapting to different case requirements and client preferences. These tools provide starting points for building your own refined systems through experience and professional development.

Resource Framework for Consistent Excellence

- Medical record review checklists ensure systematic analysis that prevents oversight while maintaining professional credibility through thorough documentation

- Case analysis templates organize complex medical information in formats that support legal argument development and attorney decision-making

- Contract templates protect consultant interests while establishing clear service relationships and professional boundary management

- Marketing materials examples provide frameworks for professional presentation that communicate qualifications effectively to attorney audiences

- Expert witness preparation guides ensure systematic readiness for testimony challenges while building confidence for effective courtroom performance

Appendix B: Technology Resources

Technology mastery represents the difference between struggling consultants who fight their tools and successful practitioners who harness technology to amplify their expertise and streamline their operations. You need systematic approaches to technology selection, implementation, and security that support practice growth while maintaining professional standards and client confidentiality.

The rapid evolution of legal and healthcare technology creates both opportunities and challenges that require ongoing evaluation and adaptation. Smart technology choices compound over time, creating competitive advantages and operational efficiency that separate successful practices from those that struggle with outdated methods.

Software Recommendations and Reviews

Case Management Systems provide the organizational backbone for professional consulting practices, enabling systematic case tracking, document management, and client communication that supports growth while maintaining quality standards.

CaseMap from LexisNexis offers litigation-specific features including timeline development, fact organization, and relationship mapping that legal professionals understand and appreciate[72]. The software integrates with other LexisNexis products while providing collaboration features for team-based case development.

Strengths include robust analytical tools, excellent attorney integration, and proven track record in litigation support. Limitations involve higher cost structure and learning curve that may exceed needs for smaller consulting practices.

MasterFile specializes in legal nurse consulting workflows with medical terminology databases, care standard references, and report templates designed specifically for healthcare litigation[73]. The system includes integrated medical references and billing features tailored to consultant needs.

Benefits include LNC-specific features, medical integration, and specialized templates. Drawbacks include limited general business features and smaller user community compared to mainstream case management systems.

Alternative Solutions for smaller practices include general business systems like Monday.com or Asana that provide project management capabilities at lower costs while offering flexibility for different practice models and growth patterns.

Document Management Platforms enable systematic organization and retrieval of medical records, research materials, and case deliverables while maintaining security and version control.

Adobe Acrobat Pro remains essential for legal document manipulation, annotation, and security features required for medical record analysis and professional report preparation[74]. Advanced features include redaction tools, digital signatures, and collaborative annotation capabilities.

Box for Business provides HIPAA-compliant cloud storage with granular access controls, audit trails, and integration capabilities that support secure case file management and client collaboration[75].

Microsoft 365 Government offers familiar productivity tools with enhanced security and compliance features appropriate for protected health information handling and professional service delivery[76].

Former emergency medicine nurse Dr. Robert Kim evaluated multiple case management solutions before selecting a hybrid approach that combined specialized LNC software with mainstream business tools for optimal functionality and cost-effectiveness.

Robert's technology stack included MasterFile for case analysis and medical record organization, QuickBooks for financial management, and Microsoft 365 for general business operations and client communication.

His integrated approach provided specialized LNC functionality while maintaining cost control and system reliability. The hybrid solution avoided vendor lock-in while providing flexibility for future growth and technology evolution.

Communication and Collaboration Tools enable effective client interaction and professional presentation while maintaining security and confidentiality requirements for legal consulting practice.

Zoom for Government provides secure video conferencing with enhanced security features appropriate for attorney-client privileged communications and expert witness preparation[77].

Microsoft Teams Government offers integrated communication, file sharing, and collaboration features within secure government-grade infrastructure that meets legal industry security requirements[78].

ProtonMail delivers end-to-end encrypted email communication that protects confidential case discussions and sensitive client information from unauthorized access or interception[79].

Cost-Benefit Analysis Worksheets

Technology Investment Evaluation Framework helps prioritize technology spending based on practice needs, expected benefits, and return on investment calculations that justify expense and guide implementation decisions.

Investment Analysis Categories:

1. **Essential Operations** - Technology required for basic practice function

2. **Efficiency Improvements** - Tools that reduce time investment or improve quality

3. **Competitive Advantages** - Systems that differentiate services or capabilities

4. **Growth Enablers** - Technology that supports practice expansion or new services

5. **Risk Management** - Security and compliance tools that protect practice and clients

ROI Calculation Methods provide systematic approaches to technology investment evaluation that consider both quantifiable benefits and strategic value for practice development.

Quantifiable Benefits Assessment:

- Time savings calculated at hourly billing rates

- Cost reductions from eliminated services or reduced overhead

- Revenue increases from improved capacity or new service capabilities

- Error reduction value calculated from prevented problems

- Client satisfaction improvements leading to referral generation

Implementation Cost Analysis includes initial purchase prices, training requirements, ongoing subscription fees, maintenance costs, and potential switching costs for technology decisions.

Hidden Cost Identification addresses training time, data migration, system integration, and productivity disruption during implementation phases that affect total technology investment value.

Former critical care nurse Dr. Patricia Thompson developed systematic technology evaluation processes that helped her make strategic investments while avoiding expensive mistakes common in early practice development.

Patricia's evaluation framework included detailed cost-benefit analysis for each technology decision, pilot testing periods for major investments, and systematic review of technology performance against expected benefits.

Her disciplined approach prevented costly mistakes while ensuring technology investments supported practice growth and competitive positioning rather than creating unnecessary complexity or expense.

Security and Compliance Guidelines

HIPAA Compliance Requirements for legal nurse consultants include technical safeguards, administrative procedures, and physical security measures that protect patient health information throughout the consulting process[80].

Technical Safeguards Implementation:

- Encryption for data at rest and in transit using AES-256 or equivalent standards

- Access controls that limit PHI access to authorized personnel only

- Audit trails that track all PHI access and modification activities

- Automatic logoff for unattended workstations and mobile devices

- Data backup and recovery procedures that maintain PHI security

Administrative Safeguards Requirements:

- Written policies and procedures for PHI handling and protection

- Workforce training on HIPAA requirements and compliance procedures

- Business associate agreements with all vendors handling PHI

- Incident response procedures for potential security breaches

- Regular risk assessments and compliance monitoring activities

Physical Safeguards Standards:

- Secure storage for physical documents containing PHI

- Workstation security measures and access controls

- Media disposal procedures for devices containing PHI

- Facility access controls and visitor management procedures

- Equipment controls for devices that process or store PHI

Cybersecurity Best Practices protect against evolving threats including ransomware, phishing attacks, and data breaches that could compromise client information and practice operations.

Network Security Measures:

- Business-grade firewall with intrusion detection capabilities

- Virtual Private Network (VPN) for remote access to practice systems

- Regular software updates and security patch management

- Endpoint protection on all devices accessing practice systems

- Network monitoring and threat detection systems

Password and Authentication Security:

- Multi-factor authentication for all business-critical systems

- Strong password requirements with regular change schedules

- Password manager usage to avoid reuse and weak passwords

- Privileged account management and access control

- Regular security awareness training for all practice personnel

Former obstetric nurse Dr. Jennifer Martinez implemented systematic security measures after a colleague's practice suffered a ransomware attack that disrupted operations and compromised client relationships.

Jennifer's security implementation included comprehensive cyber insurance, regular data backups stored offline, employee security training, and incident response procedures that protected her practice during subsequent attempted attacks.

Her proactive security approach prevented business disruption while building client confidence in her professional data handling and security practices.

Mobile App Recommendations

Productivity Applications enable effective practice management and client service delivery through mobile devices while maintaining security and professional standards for remote work capabilities.

Time Tracking Apps including Toggl, RescueTime, and Clockify provide accurate billing documentation while offering project management features that support multiple case management and client billing requirements[81].

Communication Apps like Signal, Wickr, and encrypted messaging platforms provide secure client communication capabilities that maintain confidentiality while enabling responsive service delivery[82].

Medical Reference Apps including Epocrates, Lexicomp, and UpToDate mobile versions provide instant access to medical information needed for case analysis and client consultation[83].

Document Management Apps from Box, Dropbox Business, and Microsoft OneDrive enable secure document access and collaboration while maintaining HIPAA compliance and professional security standards[84].

Financial Management Apps including QuickBooks Mobile, FreshBooks, and Wave Accounting provide invoice management, expense tracking, and financial reporting capabilities for mobile practice management[85].

VPN Applications like ExpressVPN, NordLayer, and Cisco AnyConnect provide secure internet access for remote work while protecting client confidentiality and practice security[86].

Your Technology Advantage

Technology mastery creates multiplicative advantages that compound over time, enabling efficiency improvements and competitive capabilities that separate successful consultants from those struggling with outdated methods. Your investment in learning and implementing appropriate technology systems pays dividends through improved service delivery and practice scalability.

The key lies in systematic evaluation and implementation rather than adopting every new tool or following technology trends without strategic purpose. Build technology capabilities that support your specific practice goals while maintaining security and professional standards.

Technology Success Strategies for Professional Excellence

- Software selection requires systematic evaluation of case management, document handling, and communication tools that support practice goals and client needs

- Cost-benefit analysis frameworks help prioritize technology investments based on quantifiable returns and strategic value for practice development

- Security and compliance guidelines ensure HIPAA protection and cybersecurity measures that protect client information and practice reputation

- Mobile applications enable productive remote work while maintaining professional standards and secure client communication capabilities

Appendix C: Professional Development Resources

Professional development in legal nurse consulting requires strategic navigation through multiple professional communities that often have conflicting priorities, different qualification standards, and varying approaches to knowledge validation. You need systematic approaches to continuing education that build credibility across both nursing and legal professional environments while maintaining currency with rapidly changing practice standards.

The most successful consultants build professional development portfolios that demonstrate expertise depth while showcasing ongoing learning and adaptation to industry changes. This requires understanding the different value systems and recognition patterns in healthcare and legal communities.

Certification Program Comparisons

American Association of Legal Nurse Consultants (AALNC) LNCC Program represents the gold standard certification requiring 2,000 hours of legal nurse consulting experience plus comprehensive examination covering legal concepts, healthcare standards, and professional practice[87].

The LNCC certification requires substantial experience investment before eligibility, creating the classic catch-22 where you need experience to get certified but need certification to get experience. However, LNCC recognition by attorneys and healthcare organizations provides maximum professional credibility.

Examination content includes legal system fundamentals, healthcare quality standards, research methodology, professional ethics, and business practice management. The test requires extensive preparation and demonstrates thorough knowledge across multiple professional domains.

National Alliance of Certified Legal Nurse Consultants (CLNC) Program offers more accessible entry requirements without experience prerequisites, focusing on practical skills development through intensive training programs rather than experience validation[88].

CLNC certification can be completed in weeks rather than years, making it attractive for nurses seeking immediate career transition. The program emphasizes business development, marketing, and case analysis techniques through hands-on training approaches.

However, CLNC recognition varies among legal professionals, with some preferring the more rigorous LNCC credential. The marketing-heavy approach of some CLNC programs also creates skepticism among traditional healthcare professionals.

Specialty Nursing Certifications often provide more credibility with attorney clients than general legal nurse consulting credentials because they demonstrate specialized clinical expertise relevant to specific case types[89].

Critical Care Certification (CCRN) from AACN demonstrates expertise in intensive care nursing that applies directly to critical care malpractice cases. Emergency Nursing Certification (CEN) provides credibility for trauma and emergency medicine litigation.

These specialty certifications require ongoing clinical experience and continuing education that maintains current knowledge about clinical practice standards and emerging healthcare technologies.

Former surgical nurse Dr. Sandra Chen strategically pursued multiple certifications to maximize professional recognition while building specialized expertise that commanded premium compensation.

Sandra's certification portfolio included CNOR surgical nursing certification to maintain clinical credibility, LNCC certification for legal nurse consulting recognition, and additional training in robotic surgery technology that created specialized expertise.

Her systematic approach to certification provided credibility across multiple professional communities while building competitive advantages through specialized knowledge that few consultants possessed.

University-Based Certificate Programs provide academic credentials and structured learning environments but often lack practical application focus and attorney recognition compared to professional certifications[90].

Programs from major universities offer academic rigor and comprehensive curricula but may not address practical consulting skills needed for successful practice development. Costs typically exceed professional certification programs while requiring longer time commitments.

Professional Development Planning requires understanding different certification values, cost-benefit analysis, and strategic timing for maximum career benefit and professional recognition.

Continuing Education Providers

Professional Association Programs offer continuing education specifically designed for legal nurse consultants with content addressing both clinical updates and legal industry developments.

AALNC Educational Programs include annual conferences, webinar series, and local chapter presentations that provide networking opportunities while meeting continuing education requirements for certification maintenance[91].

Annual conferences feature attorney speakers, case study presentations, and professional development sessions that address current industry trends and practice challenges. Regional programs provide local networking while offering specialized content for different practice areas.

Nursing Specialty Organizations provide clinical continuing education that maintains currency with practice standards and emerging healthcare technologies affecting litigation and expert witness requirements.

American Association of Critical-Care Nurses (AACN), Emergency Nurses Association (ENA), and specialty organizations offer clinical updates, research presentations, and practice guideline education that supports consulting credibility[92].

Legal Education Programs help consultants understand litigation processes, legal requirements, and courtroom procedures that improve consulting effectiveness and expert witness performance.

Bar association continuing education programs welcome healthcare professionals and provide education about legal processes, evidence rules, and professional requirements for expert witnesses[93].

Online Education Platforms offer flexible learning options that accommodate consulting practice schedules while providing access to specialized content and expert instruction.

Coursera, edX, and professional platforms provide courses in statistics, research methods, and specialized medical topics that support consulting competence and credibility building[94].

Former emergency medicine nurse Dr. Michael Rodriguez developed systematic continuing education plans that balanced clinical currency with legal sophistication while managing time and cost investments effectively.

Michael's education portfolio included annual emergency medicine conferences for clinical updates, quarterly legal education programs for industry knowledge, and monthly webinars addressing specific consulting challenges.

His systematic approach ensured knowledge currency while building professional networks and maintaining certification requirements across multiple professional communities.

University Partnerships with nursing schools and law schools provide access to advanced education while building academic relationships that support consulting practice and professional recognition.

Corporate Training Programs from healthcare organizations, medical device companies, and pharmaceutical firms offer specialized education about emerging technologies and their litigation implications.

Professional Associations and Benefits

American Association of Legal Nurse Consultants (AALNC) provides the primary professional home for legal nurse consultants with educational resources, networking opportunities, and advocacy for profession advancement[95].

AALNC membership includes access to professional journals, continuing education programs, networking events, and practice resources that support professional development and business growth.

Local chapters offer regular meetings, educational programs, and networking opportunities that build professional relationships while providing mentorship and practice guidance.

State Nursing Associations maintain connections with nursing professional community while providing continuing education, advocacy, and practice guidance that supports nursing license maintenance and professional credibility[96].

Many state associations include special interest groups for legal nurse consultants or alternative career paths that provide targeted resources and networking opportunities.

Bar Associations welcome healthcare professionals as associate members, providing access to legal education, networking opportunities, and professional development that builds relationships with potential clients[97].

Medical-legal committees, continuing education programs, and networking events provide opportunities to build relationships with attorneys while demonstrating expertise and professional competence.

Specialty Medical Organizations relevant to consulting practice areas provide clinical education, research access, and professional networking that supports specialized expertise development and credibility building.

Benefits Analysis for Association Membership:

- Educational resources and continuing education opportunities

- Professional networking and mentorship access

- Practice resources including templates, guidelines, and tools

- Advocacy for profession advancement and recognition

- Credibility enhancement through professional affiliation

- Business development opportunities through networking and referrals

Former pediatric nurse Dr. Lisa Park strategically leveraged multiple professional associations to build comprehensive networks that supported practice development while providing diverse educational and networking opportunities.

Lisa's association portfolio included AALNC for legal nurse consulting resources, state pediatric nursing organization for clinical currency, and local bar association for attorney networking.

Her systematic networking approach generated referrals, educational opportunities, and professional recognition that exceeded the cost of membership while building sustainable competitive advantages.

Recommended Reading and Research Sources

Legal Nurse Consulting Literature provides foundational knowledge and ongoing professional development through books, journals, and professional publications that address practice standards and industry trends.

Essential Textbooks include "Legal Nurse Consulting Principles and Practices" as comprehensive reference, "The Legal Nurse Consultant's Handbook" for practical guidance, and specialty texts addressing specific practice areas[98].

Professional Journals including Journal of Legal Nurse Consulting, AALNC publications, and legal medicine journals provide ongoing education about case studies, practice developments, and industry trends[99].

Legal Publications help consultants understand litigation processes, legal requirements, and attorney perspectives on expert witnesses and consulting services.

American Bar Association publications, state bar journals, and legal education materials provide insights into legal practice and attorney expectations for consulting services[100].

Medical Literature maintains clinical currency through specialty journals, research publications, and clinical guidelines that support expert testimony and consulting credibility.

PubMed searches, Cochrane Reviews, and specialty organization guidelines provide evidence-based information supporting case analysis and expert opinions[101].

Business and Professional Development Resources support practice management, marketing effectiveness, and professional growth through general business literature and professional service guidance.

Books on consulting practice, small business management, and professional service marketing provide strategies for practice development and client relationship management[102].

Research Database Access through professional associations, university libraries, and subscription services provides access to medical literature, legal databases, and professional resources.

LexisNexis, Westlaw, and medical databases provide research capabilities that support case analysis while building credibility through thorough preparation and current knowledge[103].

Your Learning Foundation

Professional development represents ongoing investment in your most important asset—your expertise and credibility. The systematic approach to learning and credential building separates successful consultants from those who struggle with professional recognition and competitive positioning.

Your commitment to continuous learning demonstrates professional excellence while building the knowledge base and professional relationships that support long-term practice success and industry leadership.

Professional Development Framework for Career Excellence

- Certification program selection requires understanding different credential values and strategic timing for maximum professional recognition and career benefit

- Continuing education providers offer diverse learning opportunities that should align with practice goals while maintaining clinical currency and legal sophistication

- Professional association participation provides networking, education, and advocacy benefits that exceed membership costs through relationship building and practice development

- Recommended reading and research sources maintain knowledge currency while building evidence-based analysis capabilities that support expert credibility and professional excellence

Appendix D: Financial Planning Tools

Financial management for legal nurse consulting practices requires different approaches than traditional employment because of irregular income patterns, business expense obligations, and tax considerations that employed nurses never encounter. You need systematic financial planning tools that provide stability during income fluctuations while maximizing tax advantages and building long-term financial security.

Most consultants approach financial planning with the same casual attention they'd give to weekend plans—yet financial mismanagement destroys more consulting practices than clinical incompetence or client relationship problems. Professional financial planning creates the foundation for sustainable practice growth and personal financial security.

Pricing Calculators and Worksheets

Hourly Rate Calculation Framework helps establish competitive pricing while ensuring profitability and sustainability for different service types and client arrangements.

Base Rate Calculation Method:

1. Annual income goal divided by billable hours available

2. Add overhead costs including insurance, technology, and professional development

3. Include profit margin for business growth and risk management

4. Compare with market rates for similar services and expertise levels

5. Adjust for specialization premium and competitive positioning

Market Research Components for rate validation include competitor analysis, client budget assessment, and value proposition evaluation that justifies pricing decisions.

Regional rate variations affect pricing decisions, with major metropolitan markets typically supporting higher rates than rural areas. However, remote work capabilities enable access to premium markets regardless of consultant location.

Service-Specific Pricing Strategies recognize different value propositions and market conditions for various consulting activities and client arrangements.

Medical record review rates typically range from $100-150 per hour for routine analysis, while expert witness services command $250-400 per hour for preparation and testimony time.

Specialized expertise in emerging technologies, complex medical devices, or rare conditions justifies premium pricing above standard market rates due to limited competition and specialized knowledge requirements.

Former critical care nurse Dr. Jennifer Martinez developed systematic pricing strategies that balanced competitive positioning with profitability goals while recognizing different value propositions for various service offerings.

Jennifer's pricing structure included base rates for routine case analysis, premium rates for urgent deadlines, and expert witness rates that reflected her specialized qualifications and courtroom experience.

Her systematic approach included annual rate reviews, market analysis, and value proposition assessment that justified pricing decisions while maintaining competitive positioning and client satisfaction.

Project-Based Pricing Calculations for fixed-fee services require accurate time estimation, scope definition, and risk assessment that protect profitability while providing client cost certainty.

Retainer Pricing Models provide income stability while ensuring consultant availability for client needs and urgent consulting requirements throughout extended time periods.

Rush Service Premiums compensate for schedule disruption and expedited delivery requirements while maintaining quality standards during compressed timelines.

Business Plan Templates

Executive Summary Framework for legal nurse consulting practices provides systematic business planning that addresses unique challenges and opportunities in consulting service delivery.

Business Overview Components:

- Service description and target market identification

- Competitive analysis and differentiation strategies

- Financial projections and growth planning

- Marketing strategies and client acquisition plans

- Operational procedures and quality management systems

- Risk assessment and mitigation planning

Market Analysis Section examines local litigation patterns, attorney practices, and competitive situations that affect practice viability and growth potential.

Geographic market assessment includes population demographics, healthcare system characteristics, litigation activity levels, and competitive intensity that influence practice success.

Financial Planning Components address startup costs, operating expenses, revenue projections, and cash flow management that ensure practice sustainability and growth.

Startup Cost Analysis includes technology investments, professional development, insurance requirements, and initial marketing expenses that establish practice operations.

Operating Expense Planning addresses ongoing costs including professional liability insurance, technology subscriptions, continuing education, and professional association memberships.

Revenue Projection Methods estimate income potential based on market analysis, service pricing, and capacity planning that supports financial planning and business decisions.

Former emergency medicine nurse Dr. Robert Kim developed business planning frameworks that helped him transition from employment to successful independent practice through systematic planning and financial management.

Robert's business plan included detailed market analysis of local emergency medicine litigation, competitive assessment of existing consultants, and financial projections based on conservative assumptions about case acquisition and income development.

His systematic planning approach enabled successful practice launch while avoiding common financial mistakes that undermine new consulting businesses during early development phases.

Growth Planning Strategies address practice expansion through additional services, geographic markets, or team development that increase capacity and revenue potential.

Exit Strategy Planning considers practice valuation, succession options, and transition planning that preserve practice value while providing retirement or career change flexibility.

Tax Deduction Checklists

Business Expense Categories for legal nurse consulting practices include numerous deductible expenses that reduce tax obligations while supporting practice development and professional growth.

Home Office Deductions allow consultants working from home to deduct portions of housing costs including mortgage interest, property taxes, utilities, and maintenance expenses based on exclusive business use.

Simplified home office deduction allows $5 per square foot up to 300 square feet, while actual expense method might provide larger deductions for qualifying home offices with detailed record-keeping.

Professional Development Expenses include conference attendance, certification programs, continuing education, and professional association memberships that maintain competence and build credentials.

Travel expenses for professional conferences, client meetings, and educational programs qualify for deduction when properly documented with business purpose and expense receipts.

Technology and Equipment Deductions cover computer purchases, software licenses, office furniture, and communication equipment necessary for business operations and service delivery.

Section 179 depreciation rules allow immediate expense deduction for qualifying equipment purchases up to annual limits, providing tax benefits during purchase years.

Professional Service Expenses include attorney fees, accounting services, professional consultations, and expert advice that support business operations and compliance requirements.

Former obstetric nurse Dr. Patricia Thompson maximized tax deductions through systematic expense tracking and professional tax planning that reduced her tax obligations while supporting practice growth.

Patricia's deduction strategy included home office qualification for actual expense deduction, systematic documentation of all business expenses, and strategic timing of equipment purchases for maximum tax benefit.

Her professional tax preparation included quarterly reviews with a CPA specializing in professional service businesses, ensuring compliance while maximizing legitimate deductions and tax advantages.

Quarterly Tax Planning helps consultants manage tax obligations through estimated payments and strategic expense timing that avoids penalties while optimizing cash flow.

Retirement Plan Contributions for self-employed consultants including SEP-IRA and Solo 401k options provide tax deductions while building long-term financial security.

Health Insurance Deductions for self-employed consultants allow deduction of health insurance premiums as business expenses rather than itemized deductions subject to income limitations.

Insurance Requirement Guides

Professional Liability Insurance provides essential protection against claims that consulting services caused client harm through errors, omissions, or professional negligence.

Coverage amounts typically range from $1-2 million per occurrence with annual aggregate limits that provide financial protection against litigation costs and damage awards.

Legal nurse consulting policies differ from standard nursing malpractice insurance by covering business consulting activities, expert witness testimony, and professional advice beyond direct patient care.

General Business Liability Insurance protects against premises liability, business personal property damage, and general business risks unrelated to professional services.

Cyber Liability Coverage addresses data breaches, ransomware attacks, and technology failures that could compromise protected health information or disrupt business operations.

HIPAA compliance requirements make cyber coverage increasingly important for consultants handling medical records and confidential client information.

Business Interruption Insurance replaces lost income during periods when business operations are disrupted by covered events including cyber attacks, natural disasters, or equipment failures.

Former surgical nurse Dr. Michael Rodriguez learned insurance importance through colleague experiences with professional liability claims and cyber security incidents that threatened practice viability.

Michael's insurance portfolio included professional liability coverage with expert witness protection, cyber liability insurance with business interruption coverage, and general business insurance for office operations.

His systematic insurance approach protected his practice during a frivolous malpractice claim that required extensive legal defense while allowing business continuation without financial disruption.

Workers' Compensation Requirements vary by state for consultants employing staff members, requiring compliance with local regulations and coverage requirements.

Business Auto Insurance covers vehicle use for business purposes including client meetings, deposition attendance, and professional travel activities.

Disability Insurance provides income replacement if illness or injury prevents consulting work, protecting personal financial security during health challenges.

Building Financial Security

Financial planning provides the foundation for sustainable consulting practice while protecting against the risks and uncertainties inherent in professional service businesses. Systematic financial management creates stability and growth potential that supports both business success and personal financial security.

Your commitment to professional financial planning demonstrates business sophistication while creating the financial foundation that enables practice growth and competitive positioning in demanding professional markets.

Financial Management Framework for Practice Success

- Pricing calculators and worksheets ensure competitive positioning while maintaining profitability through systematic rate development and market analysis

- Business plan templates provide strategic frameworks that address unique consulting challenges while building sustainable growth and competitive advantages

- Tax deduction checklists maximize legitimate business expense deductions while ensuring compliance with self-employment tax obligations and business requirements

- Insurance requirement guides protect against professional liability, cyber security, and business risks that could destroy practice value and personal financial security

Closing Remark

The journey from bedside nurse to successful legal nurse consultant represents more than career change—it's professional transformation that honors your clinical expertise while opening new horizons for intellectual growth, financial independence, and meaningful contribution to justice. You possess the clinical knowledge that attorneys desperately need, but success requires more than nursing expertise alone.

This handbook provides the roadmap, but your commitment to learning, professional development, and systematic practice building determines the destination. The legal nurse consulting field offers extraordinary opportunities for those willing to invest in the skills, relationships, and business acumen that separate successful consultants from those who struggle.

The attorneys who become your clients need your expertise to understand complex medical issues that determine case outcomes and client justice. Your role extends beyond case analysis to bridge the gap between medical reality and legal requirements, ensuring that healthcare accountability serves both individual clients and public safety.

Your success as a legal nurse consultant contributes to a larger mission—improving healthcare quality through professional accountability, protecting patients through expert analysis of care failures, and ensuring that justice systems understand the medical complexities they must evaluate. This work matters not just for your professional satisfaction and financial success, but for the patients whose care will improve because of the standards you help establish and maintain.

The tools, templates, and strategies in these appendices provide the operational foundation for professional excellence. Use them as starting points for developing your own refined approaches through experience and continuous improvement. Your commitment to systematic quality, professional development, and ethical practice honors both your nursing heritage and your legal consulting future.

Success in this field requires patience, persistence, and professional excellence that builds over time. The most successful legal nurse consultants combine clinical expertise with business acumen, professional relationships with technical skills, and analytical rigor with practical wisdom that serves clients and supports justice.

Your journey starts with the first case, but your legacy builds through years of professional excellence that establishes you as a trusted expert whose opinions influence important decisions about healthcare accountability and patient protection. The investment you make in building this practice creates not just personal success, but professional contribution that extends far beyond individual consulting engagements.

The future of healthcare depends partly on professionals like you who understand both clinical realities and legal requirements, who can analyze complex cases objectively, and who can communicate medical concepts clearly to legal audiences. Your work as a legal nurse consultant contributes to healthcare quality improvement while building a practice that provides both professional satisfaction and financial independence.

Essential Resource Summary for Professional Excellence

These appendices provide the operational tools and strategic guidance that successful legal nurse consultants use to build sustainable practices while maintaining professional excellence. The templates, checklists, and analytical frameworks represent accumulated wisdom from practitioners who learned through experience what works in real-world consulting situations.

Your success depends on adapting these resources to your specific practice needs while maintaining the systematic approaches that ensure quality and protect professional credibility. Professional excellence in legal nurse consulting requires both clinical expertise and business sophistication that builds over time through continuous learning and systematic improvement.

Appendix E: Geographic Market Analysis

Geographic location profoundly affects legal nurse consulting opportunities, compensation levels, and competitive intensity in ways that most nurses never consider when planning career transitions. You need systematic approaches to market evaluation that identify high-opportunity locations while understanding regulatory requirements and competitive conditions that affect practice success.

The most profitable consulting markets often exist in unexpected locations where litigation activity exceeds consultant availability, creating premium pricing opportunities for practitioners willing to serve underserved markets through strategic positioning or remote service delivery.

State-by-State Opportunity Assessment

High-Opportunity States based on malpractice claim volume, settlement values, and consultant-to-attorney ratios provide the most favorable conditions for legal nurse consulting practice development and revenue generation.

New York leads malpractice activity with $372.39 million in total payouts across 659 claims annually, creating substantial demand for expert analysis and consultation services[104]. The complex healthcare system and high damage awards justify premium consulting fees while providing numerous case opportunities.

Average compensation for legal nurse consultants in New York reaches $91,272 annually for employed positions, while independent consultants command $200-300 per hour for specialized expertise in complex metropolitan healthcare litigation.

Florida demonstrates the highest claim volume with 670 malpractice cases annually, though individual settlement amounts average lower than New York[105]. The state's large population, extensive healthcare system, and retirement community create diverse case opportunities requiring specialized geriatric and long-term care expertise.

California offers premium compensation and sophisticated litigation requiring advanced expertise in medical technology, pharmaceutical cases, and complex healthcare delivery systems that create opportunities for specialized consultants.

Texas provides substantial market opportunity through large population, extensive medical centers, and growing litigation activity that exceeds consultant availability in many metropolitan areas.

Washington leads consultant compensation with average annual salaries reaching $96,429 for employed positions while offering premium rates for independent consultants serving the technology-influenced healthcare market[106].

Emerging Opportunity States including North Carolina, Georgia, and Colorado show growing litigation activity and healthcare system expansion that create opportunities for early market entry and competitive positioning.

Former ICU nurse Dr. Patricia Martinez strategically relocated from rural Montana to Seattle to capture higher compensation opportunities while building specialized expertise in technology-enhanced critical care litigation.

Patricia's market analysis revealed Washington's premium compensation, growing technology litigation, and limited competition from consultants with her critical care background and technology expertise.

Her strategic relocation resulted in 40% income increase during the first year while providing access to complex cases involving medical technology that weren't available in her rural market.

Market Saturation Analysis helps identify locations where consultant supply exceeds demand, creating competitive pressure and pricing constraints that limit practice growth and profitability.

Rural Market Opportunities often provide less competition and closer attorney relationships but may offer limited case volume and lower compensation due to smaller damage awards and budget constraints.

Metropolitan Market Challenges include higher competition, increased overhead costs, and more sophisticated client expectations while offering premium compensation and complex case opportunities.

Salary and Rate Benchmarks

Regional Compensation Variations reflect local market conditions, cost of living differences, and litigation activity levels that affect both employed and independent consultant earning potential.

Employed Position Compensation ranges from $45,000 in rural markets to $96,000 in premium metropolitan areas, with benefits packages and advancement opportunities varying significantly between markets and employers[107].

Insurance companies typically offer lower base salaries but provide comprehensive benefits, regular hours, and advancement opportunities through claims management and senior review positions.

Law firms generally provide higher compensation but may require longer hours, variable workload, and performance-based compensation tied to case outcomes and client satisfaction.

Independent Consultant Rates vary from $100-150 per hour in competitive or rural markets to $250-400 per hour for specialized expertise in premium metropolitan markets.

Expert witness rates consistently exceed consulting rates, with testimony commanding $250-400 per hour plus travel time and preparation fees regardless of geographic location.

Specialization Premium affects compensation across all markets, with consultants possessing expertise in emerging technologies, rare conditions, or specialized procedures commanding rates 25-50% above general practice levels.

Former emergency medicine nurse Dr. Michael Rodriguez analyzed geographic compensation patterns before establishing his practice location and service delivery model to maximize earning potential.

Michael's analysis revealed that remote service delivery enabled access to premium metropolitan rates while maintaining lower rural overhead costs, creating optimal financial positioning.

His virtual practice model served attorneys in major metropolitan markets while operating from a lower-cost rural location, resulting in effective hourly rates exceeding $200 while maintaining lifestyle preferences.

Market Entry Strategies for different geographic areas require understanding local attorney practices, referral patterns, and competitive positioning that affect practice development and client acquisition.

Cost of Living Adjustments must be considered when evaluating compensation opportunities, as higher nominal rates in expensive markets may provide lower real income than moderate rates in affordable locations.

Licensing and Regulatory Requirements

Nursing License Requirements vary by state and affect consultant qualifications, continuing education obligations, and practice scope for legal nurse consulting activities.

Multi-State Licensing Compacts enable practice across state lines for consultants licensed in compact states, expanding market access while simplifying regulatory compliance for multi-state consulting practices[108].

Continuing Education Requirements differ significantly between states, ranging from 15-30 hours annually with varying requirements for specialty areas, ethics training, and pharmacology education.

Professional Practice Requirements including scope of practice limitations, supervision requirements, and professional responsibility standards affect consulting capabilities and expert witness qualification.

Business Registration Requirements for consulting practices vary by state and include business licensing, professional registration, and tax compliance obligations that affect practice establishment and operation.

Professional Liability Insurance requirements differ between states, with some requiring specific coverage amounts or policy features for healthcare professionals providing consulting services.

Former surgical nurse Dr. Jennifer Williams researched multi-state practice requirements before establishing her practice to serve clients across multiple jurisdictions while maintaining compliance with all regulatory requirements.

Jennifer's compliance strategy included nursing license compact participation, professional liability insurance meeting all state requirements, and business registration in her primary practice state.

Her systematic approach to regulatory compliance enabled multi-state practice while avoiding legal complications that could affect client relationships or professional standing.

Telehealth Practice Regulations increasingly affect legal nurse consultants providing remote services across state lines, requiring understanding of emerging regulatory frameworks and compliance requirements[109].

Professional Corporation Requirements in some states mandate specific business structures for licensed healthcare professionals providing consulting services.

Continuing Education Reciprocity between states affects professional development planning and compliance costs for consultants practicing across multiple jurisdictions.

Professional Association Contacts

American Association of Legal Nurse Consultants (AALNC) maintains local chapters in major metropolitan areas that provide networking opportunities, continuing education, and professional development resources[110].

State Chapter Locations include California, Texas, Florida, New York, and other major markets with regular meetings, educational programs, and networking events that support practice development and professional relationships.

Local Chapter Benefits include peer mentorship, referral opportunities, continuing education programs, and professional recognition that support practice growth and competitive positioning.

State Nursing Associations provide professional support, continuing education, and advocacy for nursing professionals while maintaining connections with traditional nursing community[111].

Bar Association Medical-Legal Committees offer networking opportunities with attorneys while providing education about legal requirements and attorney expectations for expert witnesses and consultants[112].

Regional Professional Networks including healthcare law societies, medical professional liability organizations, and specialty bar associations provide additional networking and educational opportunities.

Professional Development Resources through state organizations include continuing education programs, certification support, and practice guidance that helps consultants navigate local market conditions and regulatory requirements.

Former critical care nurse Dr. Sandra Chen built professional networks across multiple states through systematic association participation that generated referrals and practice opportunities beyond her primary market.

Sandra's networking strategy included AALNC chapter participation in three states, bar association membership in her primary market, and specialty organization involvement that created diverse referral sources.

Her multi-state networking approach generated consulting opportunities that exceeded her individual capacity while building professional recognition across regional markets.

Contact Information Resources for professional associations include websites, membership directories, and professional publications that provide access to networking opportunities and professional development resources.

Membership Benefits Analysis helps consultants evaluate association value based on networking opportunities, educational resources, and practice development benefits relative to membership costs and time investment.

Your Geographic Strategy

Geographic market analysis provides the foundation for strategic practice development that maximizes opportunities while understanding competitive and regulatory conditions affecting consulting success. Location decisions profoundly affect earning potential, practice growth, and professional development opportunities throughout consulting careers.

Your approach to geographic positioning should balance compensation opportunities with lifestyle preferences, competitive conditions, and market growth potential that supports long-term practice success and professional satisfaction.

Geographic Market Framework for Strategic Success

- State-by-state opportunity assessment reveals high-potential markets with favorable litigation activity, compensation levels, and competitive conditions for practice development

- Salary and rate benchmarks provide realistic compensation expectations while identifying premium markets and specialization opportunities that justify strategic positioning

- Licensing and regulatory requirements affect multi-state practice capabilities while ensuring compliance with professional obligations and business registration requirements

- Professional association contacts provide networking opportunities and practice development resources that support market entry and competitive positioning across different geographic areas

Reference

1. Business Research Insights. (2024). Legal Consulting Services Market Growth Analysis Report, 2033. Retrieved from https://www.businessresearchinsights.com/market-reports/legal-consulting-services-market-122233

2. Research.com. (2025). What is a Legal Nurse Consultant: Salary & Career Paths for 2025. Retrieved from https://research.com/careers/what-is-a-legal-nurse-consultant-salary-and-career-paths

3. Legalnurse.com. (2025). 2025: Legal Nurse Consultant Jobs Outlook for Career Growth and Salaries. Retrieved from https://www.legalnurse.com/what-is-a-legal-nurse-consultant/legal-nurse-consultant-jobs-resources/legal-nurse-consultant-jobs/legal-nurse-consultant-jobs-outlook-for-career-growth-and-salaries

4. NCHStats. (2025). Medical Malpractice Payouts By State Analysis (2025). Retrieved from https://nchstats.com/medical-malpractice-payouts-by-state/

5. U.S. Bureau of Labor Statistics. (2024). Registered Nurses: Occupational Outlook Handbook. Retrieved from https://www.bls.gov/ooh/healthcare/registered-nurses.htm

6. PayScale. (2025). Legal Nurse Consultant Hourly Pay in 2025. Retrieved from https://www.payscale.com/research/US/Job=Legal_Nurse_Consultant/Hourly_Rate

7. Legalnurse.com. (2025). RN Job and Legal Nurse Consultant Salary Comparison. Retrieved from https://www.legalnurse.com/what-is-a-legal-nurse-

consultant/legal-nurse-consultant-jobs-resources/legal-nurse-consultant-salary/rn-job-and-legal-nurse-consultant-salary-comparison

8. U.S. Legal Support. (2024). RemoteDepo Pro: The Future of Remote Depositions. Retrieved from https://www.uslegalsupport.com/blog/remotedepo-pro-the-future-of-remote-depositions/

9. LNC Accelerator. (2024). The 5 Essential Legal Nurse Consulting Tools You Need to Dominate the Industry. Retrieved from https://lncaccelerator.com/the-5-essential-legal-nurse-consulting-tools-you-need-to-dominate-the-industry/

10. LNC Tips. (2024). Software to Get You Started. Retrieved from https://www.lnctips.com/software

11. Legalnurse.com. (2024). 22 Productivity Apps for Certified Legal Nurse Consultants on the Move. Retrieved from https://www.legalnurse.com/legal-nurse-consulting-blog/2019/07/22-productivity-apps-for-certified-legal-nurse-consultants-on-the-move

12. MRC Houston. (2024). The Role of AI in Legal Nurse Consulting - Revolutionizing Case Analysis in Mass Torts. Retrieved from https://mrchouston.com/the-role-of-ai-in-legal-nurse-consulting-revolutionizing-case-analysis-in-mass-torts/

13. U.S. Legal Support. (2024). RemoteDepo Pro: The Future of Remote Depositions. Retrieved from https://www.uslegalsupport.com/blog/remotedepo-pro-the-future-of-remote-depositions/

14. Legal Nurse Business. (2024). How to Start a Legal Nurse Consulting Business. Retrieved from

https://legalnursebusiness.com/how-to-start-a-legal-nurse-consulting-business/

15. LNC Accelerator. (2024). Common Challenges in Legal Nurse Consulting and How to Overcome Them. Retrieved from https://lncaccelerator.com/common-challenges-in-legal-nurse-consulting-and-how-to-overcome-them/

16. American Institute of Health Care Professionals. (2024). Legal Nurse Consulting and Malpractice. Retrieved from https://aihcp.net/2024/01/18/66384/

17. Legalnurse.com. (2024). Types of Cases Handled by Legal Nurse Consultants. Retrieved from https://www.legalnurse.com/what-is-a-legal-nurse-consultant/types-of-legal-cases

18. LNC Tips. (2024). LNC Types. Retrieved from https://www.lnctips.com/LNCTypes

19. Nurse.org. (2024). How to Become a Legal Nurse Consultant (LNC). Retrieved from https://nurse.org/resources/legal-nurse-consultant/

20. NPHub. (2024). The Essential Guide to Becoming a Nurse Practitioner Legal Consultant. Retrieved from https://www.nphub.com/blog/legal-nurse-consultant-nurse-practitioner-guide

21. University of Georgia. (2024). Legal Nurse Consultant Training from UGA Continuing Education. Retrieved from https://www.georgiacenter.uga.edu/courses/healthcare/legal-nurse-consultant-training-course

22. Loyola University. (2024). Legal Nurse Consultant. Retrieved from https://aspire.loyola.edu/products/2463529347

23. OAS Inc. (2024). What Is Medical Record Review In Legal Cases? Retrieved from https://www.oasinc.org/what-is-medical-record-review-in-legal-cases

24. LNC Tips. (2024). Information for New LNCs. Retrieved from https://www.lnctips.com/overconfident

25. LNC Stats. (2024). 7 Common Misconceptions about Becoming a Legal Nurse Consultant. Retrieved from https://www.lncstat.com/legalnurseconsultingnews/articles/2017/7-Common-Misconceptions-about-Becoming-a-Legal-Nurse-Consultant.php

26. Legalnurse.com. (2024). 5 Minimum Qualifications for How to Become a Legal Nurse Consultant. Retrieved from https://www.legalnurse.com/what-is-a-legal-nurse-consultant/legal-nurse-consultant-jobs-resources/how-to-become-a-legal-nurse-consultant/5-minimum-qualifications-for-how-to-become-a-legal-nurse-consultant

27. Legalnurse.com. (2024). 18 Common Mistakes Certified Legal Nurse Consultants Make When Launching Their CLNC Business. Retrieved from https://www.legalnurse.com/legal-nurse-consulting-blog/2019/11/18-common-mistakes-certified-legal-nurse-consultants-make-when-launching-their-clnc-business

28. Amazon. (2024). Legal Nurse Consulting Principles and Practices. Retrieved from https://www.amazon.com/Legal-Nurse-Consulting-Principles-Practices/dp/0367246406

29. Amazon. (2024). Legal Nurse Consulting: Principles and Practice, Second Edition. Retrieved from https://www.amazon.com/Legal-Nurse-Consulting-Principles-Practice/dp/0849314186

30. MasterFile. (2024). Legal Nurse Consultants. Retrieved from https://masterfile.biz/legal-nurse-consultants-lp/

31. EveryNurse. (2024). Importance of Legal Nurse Consultants in the Medical Field. Retrieved from https://everynurse.org/importance-legal-nurse-consultants-medical-legal-field/

32. American Association of Legal Nurse Consultants. (2024). LNCC Certification. Retrieved from https://lncc.aalnc.org/LNCC-Certification

33. Legal Nurse Business. (2024). How to Start a Legal Nurse Consulting Business. Retrieved from https://legalnursebusiness.com/how-to-start-a-legal-nurse-consulting-business/

34. Legalnurse.com. (2024). 18 Common Mistakes Certified Legal Nurse Consultants Make When Launching Their CLNC Business. Retrieved from https://www.legalnurse.com/legal-nurse-consulting-blog/2019/11/18-common-mistakes-certified-legal-nurse-consultants-make-when-launching-their-clnc-business

35. LNC Accelerator. (2024). Common Challenges in Legal Nurse Consulting and How to Overcome Them. Retrieved from https://lncaccelerator.com/common-challenges-in-legal-nurse-consulting-and-how-to-overcome-them/

36. LNC Tips. (2024). Information for New LNCs. Retrieved from https://www.lnctips.com/overconfident

37. Legalnurse.com. (2024). 5 Minimum Qualifications for How to Become a Legal Nurse Consultant. Retrieved from https://www.legalnurse.com/what-is-a-legal-nurse-consultant/legal-nurse-consultant-jobs-resources/how-to-

become-a-legal-nurse-consultant/5-minimum-qualifications-for-how-to-become-a-legal-nurse-consultant

38. TCK Publishing. (2024). How to Write Book Titles That Sell: 5 SEO Tips for Creating a Nonfiction Book Title. Retrieved from https://www.tckpublishing.com/how-to-write-book-titles-that-sell/

39. LNC Accelerator. (2024). The 5 Essential Legal Nurse Consulting Tools You Need to Dominate the Industry. Retrieved from https://lncaccelerator.com/the-5-essential-legal-nurse-consulting-tools-you-need-to-dominate-the-industry/

40. LNC Tips. (2024). Software to Get You Started. Retrieved from https://www.lnctips.com/software

41. Legalnurse.com. (2024). 22 Productivity Apps for Certified Legal Nurse Consultants on the Move. Retrieved from https://www.legalnurse.com/legal-nurse-consulting-blog/2019/07/22-productivity-apps-for-certified-legal-nurse-consultants-on-the-move

42. Nurse.org. (2024). How to Become a Legal Nurse Consultant (LNC). Retrieved from https://nurse.org/resources/legal-nurse-consultant/

43. Legalnurse.com. (2024). Types of Cases Handled by Legal Nurse Consultants. Retrieved from https://www.legalnurse.com/what-is-a-legal-nurse-consultant/types-of-legal-cases

44. LNC Tips. (2024). LNC Types. Retrieved from https://www.lnctips.com/LNCTypes

45. NPHub. (2024). The Essential Guide to Becoming a Nurse Practitioner Legal Consultant. Retrieved from

https://www.nphub.com/blog/legal-nurse-consultant-nurse-practitioner-guide

46. University of Georgia. (2024). Legal Nurse Consultant Training from UGA Continuing Education. Retrieved from https://www.georgiacenter.uga.edu/courses/healthcare/legal-nurse-consultant-training-course

47. Loyola University. (2024). Legal Nurse Consultant. Retrieved from https://aspire.loyola.edu/products/2463529347

48. OAS Inc. (2024). What Is Medical Record Review In Legal Cases? Retrieved from https://www.oasinc.org/what-is-medical-record-review-in-legal-cases

49. LNC Stats. (2024). 7 Common Misconceptions about Becoming a Legal Nurse Consultant. Retrieved from https://www.lncstat.com/legalnurseconsultingnews/articles/2017/7-Common-Misconceptions-about-Becoming-a-Legal-Nurse-Consultant.php

50. LNC Tips. (2024). Information for New LNCs. Retrieved from https://www.lnctips.com/overconfident

51. Legalnurse.com. (2024). 5 Minimum Qualifications for How to Become a Legal Nurse Consultant. Retrieved from https://www.legalnurse.com/what-is-a-legal-nurse-consultant/legal-nurse-consultant-jobs-resources/how-to-become-a-legal-nurse-consultant/5-minimum-qualifications-for-how-to-become-a-legal-nurse-consultant

52. Legalnurse.com. (2024). 18 Common Mistakes Certified Legal Nurse Consultants Make When Launching Their CLNC Business. Retrieved from https://www.legalnurse.com/legal-nurse-consulting-blog/2019/11/18-common-mistakes-certified-legal-nurse-consultants-make-when-launching-their-clnc-business

53. Amazon. (2024). Legal Nurse Consulting Principles and Practices. Retrieved from https://www.amazon.com/Legal-Nurse-Consulting-Principles-Practices/dp/0367246406

54. Amazon. (2024). Legal Nurse Consulting: Principles and Practice, Second Edition. Retrieved from https://www.amazon.com/Legal-Nurse-Consulting-Principles-Practice/dp/0849314186

55. LNC Accelerator. (2024). The 5 Essential Legal Nurse Consulting Tools You Need to Dominate the Industry. Retrieved from https://lncaccelerator.com/the-5-essential-legal-nurse-consulting-tools-you-need-to-dominate-the-industry/

56. MRC Houston. (2024). The Role of AI in Legal Nurse Consulting - Revolutionizing Case Analysis in Mass Torts. Retrieved from https://mrchouston.com/the-role-of-ai-in-legal-nurse-consulting-revolutionizing-case-analysis-in-mass-torts/

57. Legal Nurse Business. (2024). How to Start a Legal Nurse Consulting Business. Retrieved from https://legalnursebusiness.com/how-to-start-a-legal-nurse-consulting-business/

58. LNC Accelerator. (2024). Common Challenges in Legal Nurse Consulting and How to Overcome Them. Retrieved from https://lncaccelerator.com/common-challenges-in-legal-nurse-consulting-and-how-to-overcome-them/

59. American Institute of Health Care Professionals. (2024). Legal Nurse Consulting and Malpractice. Retrieved from https://aihcp.net/2024/01/18/66384/

60. MasterFile. (2024). Legal Nurse Consultants. Retrieved from https://masterfile.biz/legal-nurse-consultants-lp/

61. EveryNurse. (2024). Importance of Legal Nurse Consultants in the Medical Field. Retrieved from https://everynurse.org/importance-legal-nurse-consultants-medical-legal-field/

62. NPHub. (2024). The Essential Guide to Becoming a Nurse Practitioner Legal Consultant. Retrieved from https://www.nphub.com/blog/legal-nurse-consultant-nurse-practitioner-guide

63. American Association of Legal Nurse Consultants. (2024). LNCC Certification. Retrieved from https://lncc.aalnc.org/LNCC-Certification

64. TCK Publishing. (2024). How to Write Book Titles That Sell: 5 SEO Tips for Creating a Nonfiction Book Title. Retrieved from https://www.tckpublishing.com/how-to-write-book-titles-that-sell/

65. American Association of Legal Nurse Consultants. (2024). LNCC Certification - Legal Nurse Consultant Certification. Retrieved from https://lncc.aalnc.org/LNCC-Certification

66. MRC Houston. (2024). The Role of AI in Legal Nurse Consulting - Revolutionizing Case Analysis in Mass Torts. Retrieved from https://mrchouston.com/the-role-of-ai-in-legal-nurse-consulting-revolutionizing-case-analysis-in-mass-torts/

67. U.S. Legal Support. (2024). RemoteDepo Pro: The Future of Remote Depositions. Retrieved from https://www.uslegalsupport.com/blog/remotedepo-pro-the-future-of-remote-depositions/

68. Cloudester. (2024). The Future of AI Consulting: Trends and Predictions for 2025. Retrieved from

https://cloudester.com/future-of-ai-consulting-trends-and-predictions-2024/

69. LNC Accelerator. (2024). The 5 Essential Legal Nurse Consulting Tools You Need to Dominate the Industry. Retrieved from https://lncaccelerator.com/the-5-essential-legal-nurse-consulting-tools-you-need-to-dominate-the-industry/

70. LNC Accelerator. (2024). Common Challenges in Legal Nurse Consulting and How to Overcome Them. Retrieved from https://lncaccelerator.com/common-challenges-in-legal-nurse-consulting-and-how-to-overcome-them/

71. Research.com. (2025). What is a Legal Nurse Consultant: Salary & Career Paths for 2025. Retrieved from https://research.com/careers/what-is-a-legal-nurse-consultant-salary-and-career-paths

72. LexisNexis. (2024). CaseMap Legal Case Management Software. Retrieved from https://www.lexisnexis.com/en-us/products/casemap.page

73. MasterFile. (2024). Legal Nurse Consulting Software Solutions. Retrieved from https://masterfile.biz/legal-nurse-consultants-lp/

74. Adobe. (2024). Adobe Acrobat Pro for Legal Professionals. Retrieved from https://www.adobe.com/acrobat/business.html

75. Box. (2024). Box for Business - HIPAA Compliant Cloud Storage. Retrieved from https://www.box.com/business

76. Microsoft. (2024). Microsoft 365 Government Cloud Services. Retrieved from https://www.microsoft.com/en-us/microsoft-365/government

77. Zoom. (2024). Zoom for Government - Secure Video Conferencing. Retrieved from https://zoom.us/government

78. Microsoft. (2024). Microsoft Teams for Government. Retrieved from https://www.microsoft.com/en-us/microsoft-teams/government

79. ProtonMail. (2024). Secure Email for Business. Retrieved from https://proton.me/business

80. HHS.gov. (2024). HIPAA Security Rule Technical Safeguards. Retrieved from https://www.hhs.gov/hipaa/for-professionals/security/index.html

81. Toggl. (2024). Professional Time Tracking Software. Retrieved from https://toggl.com/track/

82. Signal. (2024). Secure Messaging for Business. Retrieved from https://signal.org/

83. Epocrates. (2024). Medical Reference Mobile App. Retrieved from https://www.epocrates.com/

84. Box. (2024). Mobile Document Management Apps. Retrieved from https://www.box.com/mobile

85. QuickBooks. (2024). Mobile Accounting Solutions. Retrieved from https://quickbooks.intuit.com/mobile/

86. ExpressVPN. (2024). Business VPN Solutions. Retrieved from https://www.expressvpn.com/business

87. American Association of Legal Nurse Consultants. (2024). LNCC Certification Requirements. Retrieved from https://lncc.aalnc.org/LNCC-Certification

88. National Alliance of Certified Legal Nurse Consultants. (2024). CLNC Certification Program. Retrieved from https://www.legalnurse.com/what-is-a-legal-nurse-

consultant/legal-nurse-consultant-jobs-resources/how-to-become-a-legal-nurse-consultant/5-minimum-qualifications-for-how-to-become-a-legal-nurse-consultant

89. American Association of Critical-Care Nurses. (2024). CCRN Certification. Retrieved from https://www.aacn.org/certification/get-certified/ccrn-adult

90. University of Georgia. (2024). Legal Nurse Consultant Certificate Program. Retrieved from https://www.georgiacenter.uga.edu/courses/healthcare/legal-nurse-consultant-training-course

91. American Association of Legal Nurse Consultants. (2024). Educational Programs and Resources. Retrieved from https://www.aalnc.org/

92. Emergency Nurses Association. (2024). Continuing Education Programs. Retrieved from https://www.ena.org/education

93. American Bar Association. (2024). Continuing .Legal Education Programs. Retrieved from https://www.americanbar.org/groups/continuing_legal_education/

94. Coursera. (2024). Professional Development Courses for Healthcare. Retrieved from https://www.coursera.org/browse/health

95. American Association of Legal Nurse Consultants. (2024). Membership Benefits and Resources. Retrieved from https://www.aalnc.org/membership

96. American Nurses Association. (2024). State Nursing Association Directory. Retrieved from https://www.nursingworld.org/membership/

97. American Bar Association. (2024). Associate Membership for Healthcare Professionals. Retrieved from https://www.americanbar.org/membership/

98. Amazon. (2024). Legal Nurse Consulting: Principles and Practice, Second Edition. Retrieved from https://www.amazon.com/Legal-Nurse-Consulting-Principles-Practice/dp/0849314186

99. Journal of Legal Nurse Consulting. (2024). Professional Publication for Legal Nurse Consultants. Retrieved from https://www.aalnc.org/publications

100. American Bar Association. (2024). Legal Publications and Journals. Retrieved from https://www.americanbar.org/groups/publications/

101. PubMed. (2024). Medical Literature Database. Retrieved from https://pubmed.ncbi.nlm.nih.gov/

102. Harvard Business Review. (2024). Professional Service Business Management. Retrieved from https://hbr.org/topic/professional-services

103. LexisNexis. (2024). Legal Research Database Services. Retrieved from https://www.lexisnexis.com/en-us/products/lexis-advance.page

104. NCHStats. (2025). Medical Malpractice Payouts By State Analysis (2025). Retrieved from https://nchstats.com/medical-malpractice-payouts-by-state/

105. Research.com. (2025). Legal Nurse Consultant Market Analysis by State. Retrieved from https://research.com/careers/what-is-a-legal-nurse-consultant-salary-and-career-paths

106.   PayScale. (2025). Legal Nurse Consultant Salary by Geographic Location. Retrieved from https://www.payscale.com/research/US/Job=Legal_Nurse_Consultant/Salary

107.   Legalnurse.com. (2025). Geographic Salary Comparison for Legal Nurse Consultants. Retrieved from https://www.legalnurse.com/what-is-a-legal-nurse-consultant/legal-nurse-consultant-jobs-resources/legal-nurse-consultant-salary/

108.   National Council of State Boards of Nursing. (2024). Nurse Licensure Compact Information. Retrieved from https://www.ncsbn.org/nursing-regulation/nurse-licensure-compact

109.   Federation of State Medical Boards. (2024). Telemedicine Policy and Licensing Requirements. Retrieved from https://www.fsmb.org/advocacy/telemedicine/

110.   American Association of Legal Nurse Consultants. (2024). Local Chapter Directory and Contact Information. Retrieved from https://www.aalnc.org/chapters

111.   American Nurses Association. (2024). State Nursing Association Contact Directory. Retrieved from https://www.nursingworld.org/membership/

112.   American Bar Association. (2024). Medical-Legal Committee Directory. Retrieved from https://www.americanbar.org/groups/health_law/

www.ingramcontent.com/pod-product-compliance
Lightning Source LLC
Chambersburg PA
CBHW070752270326
41927CB00010B/2122